CONTENTS

D0245321

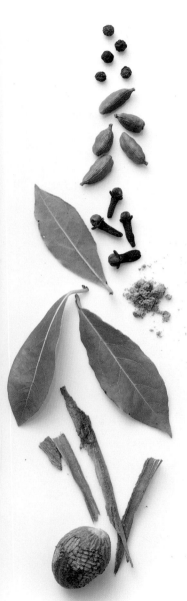

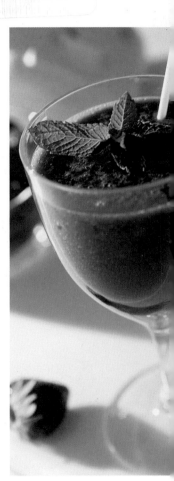

FOREWORD

Pregnancy is a time of great change and upheaval – physically, emotionally and spiritually. It is a time when the nourishment of the new life inside you is critical so you will find yourself looking more carefully at what you eat and having to take care with certain foods. Yet for some pregnant women, eating itself can be difficult for several reasons. At a time when your hormones may be making you feel nauseous anyway, the smell of cooking can be hard to take. Familiar foods may suddenly lead to heartburn, and constipation may make you reluctant to eat at all.

The importance of good nutrition in utero is without question; it has been clear for some time that what happens in those nine months is a major determinant of your baby's long-term health and what you eat and what you don't will have enormous consequences throughout his or her life. But what happens if eating proper meals is or becomes difficult? What if you can't face being in the kitchen for more than a few minutes or you just don't fancy foods or can't keep much down? Nutritious drinks may be one simple answer.

I wrote *Super Drinks for Pregnancy* to help healthy women get great nutrition throughout pregnancy. My aim was to provide a host of different recipes and ideas so that even when you can't eat as you'd like, you can still maintain a good pregnancy diet by having nutrient-packed food in liquid form, such as smoothies, juices and soups. Nor should you have to feel left out when everyone else is partying or you're in the mood for a special treat; the book contains some luscious party drinks and mocktails as well as great alternatives to your daily cups of tea or coffee.

While not intended to replace your regular diet, the drinks will boost your nutritional intake when your needs are great and your healthy intentions are thwarted by feeling nauseous, or you are just short of time or energy. They should also take the place of

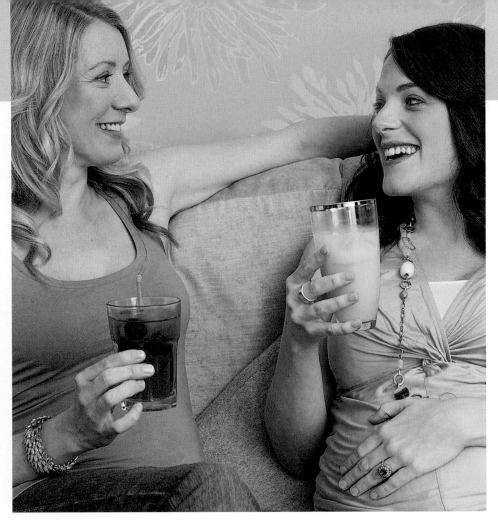

caffeinated and alcoholic beverages, which are not recommended at this special time. There are even some that may help you overcome, or at least cope with, some common pregnancy complaints.

Each of the recipes has been nutritionally analysed so you can see at a glance what it contains, how many calories it will contribute to your daily diet and how its ingredients may help you – and your baby – in pregnancy and beyond. Many of the drinks are high in valuable nutrients while all of them are simple – and fairly quick – to prepare. I hope you enjoy them!

Fiona Wilcock

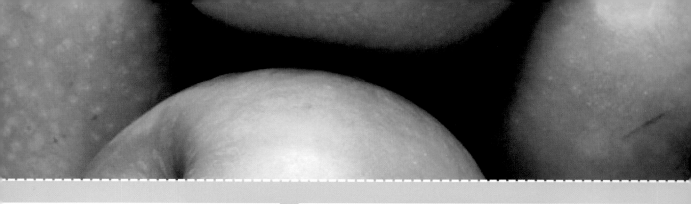
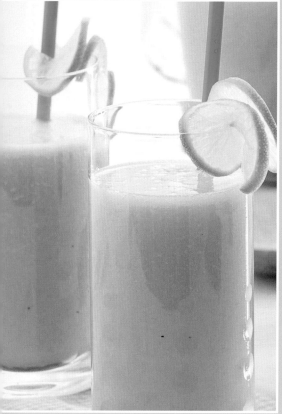
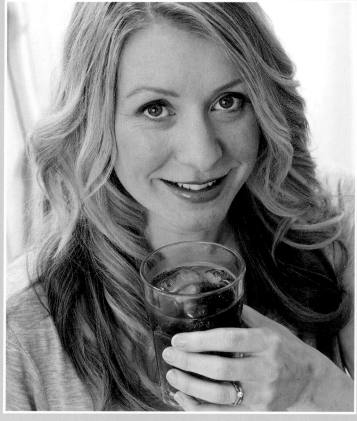
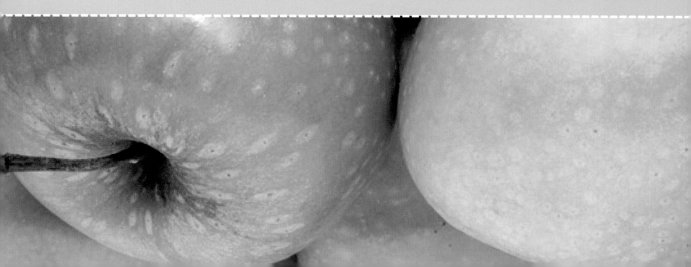

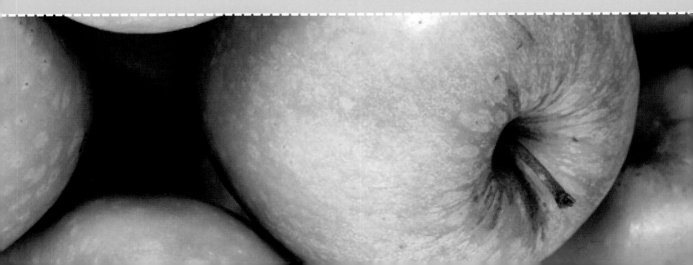

WHY FOCUS ON DRINKS?

The topic of drinks in pregnancy is often focused on the negative – what you shouldn't have, rather than what you can and should be drinking. So many women get stuck at the 'I must replace my high octane coffee with herb tea' and 'I'll have an orange juice and drive home as I'm not drinking', neither of which reflects the many positive reasons for thinking about the liquid part of our diets.

Whether you are pregnant or breastfeeding, your nutritional and hydration needs increase, and by choosing your drinks carefully you can meet both needs. This section provides you with a comprehensive background on how drinks can boost your pregnancy nutrition, and alleviate some common pregnancy complaints as well as keeping you hydrated. Prepare to focus on the positive!

The importance of hydration

ARE YOU DRINKING ENOUGH?

An easy way of knowing whether you are taking in sufficient fluids is to look at your urine. If it is a dark colour, you are not drinking enough; pale urine indicates that you are well hydrated.

Being adequately hydrated is necessary at every stage of life but during pregnancy and when you are breastfeeding, it becomes even more vital because of the many physiological changes that are taking place.

Before looking in more detail at the effect of pregnancy on the amount of fluid you need, it is important to understand the role of water in the body. The average woman is estimated to be composed of around 50% water; for a 60 kg (9st 6lb) woman, this means she contains about 33 litres (58 pints) of water. Blood contains around 83% water by weight, muscle 76% and skin 72% and even bone contains 22% water by weight. Water is not only present in the body in fluids, but it also plays an essential role in carrying compounds, gases and nutrients around the body in blood, lymph and other fluids. It is also critical to many different metabolic reactions as well as helping to keep the body at the correct temperature.

Amazingly, our bodies are able to keep the large amount of water they contain in tight control. We produce a hormone (vasopressin), which regulates our water balance; it acts on the kidneys so they produce more or less urine as required. However, water is constantly being lost – through respiration, perspiration, urination, defaecation and other bodily processes. As the body relies on maintaining a pretty constant amount of water, it is vital for good health that we take in water from foods and drinks every day to be adequately hydrated. Water loss increases if you have a fever, are exercising or are in a hot place, so hydration at these times is even more important.

HOW MUCH WATER DO YOU NEED?

Until recently there have been no internationally agreed recommendations for how much fluid is needed: the rule-of-thumb figure has generally been given as 6–8 glasses or 1.5–2 litres of water daily. In 2010, the European Food Standards Agency provided a Scientific Opinion on Dietary Reference Values for Water, which recommended that non-pregnant women need 2 litres (3½ pints) per day, while pregnant women require an additional 300 ml (in total 2.3 litres or 4 pints) and breastfeeding women an additional 600–700 ml (in total 2.6–2.7 litres or 4¾ pints). Around 70–80% of water intake should be provided by drinks and the remaining 20–30% by foods containing water (soups, fruit, vegetables, and so on).

WATER IN FOODS

Foods contain different amounts of water, all of which count toward your daily intake of 2–2.7 litres of fluids. The table (right) shows the water content of some common foods. The higher the water content in raw foods, the fewer the calories, so these foods also make ideal snacks as they won't add many calories.

HYDRATION NEEDS IN PREGNANCY AND WHEN BREASTFEEDING

It is estimated that two thirds of the weight gain of pregnancy can be attributed to water. This is accounted for by increases in blood volume; the growth of the uterus, placenta and breasts; and the development of amniotic and other fluids. On top of this is, of course, the developing baby who is composed of around 94% water by the end of the first trimester and 75% water at birth.

Blood is an important transporter of nutrients around your body, so it is not surprising that it starts to increase in volume from about the sixth week of pregnancy. By the time you have reached your 34th week, an average of an additional litre and a half of blood has been made.

The amount of amniotic fluid also increases – from almost nothing to around a litre at 38 weeks. Being properly hydrated ensures that you have adequate amniotic fluid, which protects your baby from being squashed, aids the maturation of your baby's organs and also provides a barrier against infection.

Not only do you need additional fluid to provide for the increases in your blood and amniotic fluid, but adequate hydration is necessary to ensure you don't become constipated as a result of the many circulating pregnancy hormones. Some of the hormones, which relax your muscles and ligaments, also influence those of your intestines, so food and waste is pushed less efficiently through your body. Constipation is even more of a problem in late pregnancy when your internal organs have to accommodate your increasingly large baby. Around 30% of women suffer from constipation at some stage of pregnancy, so it is important to ensure you have plenty of water and fibre and continue to be active as all of these help keep things moving along. (There are plenty of recipes in the book which contain good amounts of fibre.)

Nausea and sickness, particularly in the early months, are thought to be caused by the hormone human chorionic gonadotrophin (HCG). Although many women feel sick, not all actually vomit. Should you be one of those who can't keep food down, it is really important to replenish the lost water and salts through sipping drinks. If you are being sick several

WATER CONTENT OF COMMON FOODS

Food	% of water	Average portion g	Kilocalories in average portion	Portion of food
FRUIT AND VEGETABLES				
Apple	83	150	69	1 medium apple
Banana	75	100	95	1 small banana
Broccoli	88	85	28	3–4 florets
Carrot, raw	88	80	24	1 medium carrot
Celery	95	60	4	2 sticks celery
Mushrooms	93	50	6	Handful mushrooms
Peach	89	160	52	1 medium peach
Pear	84	160	64	1 medium pear
Strawberries	90	100	27	8–10 strawberries
Tomato	93	85	14	1 medium tomato
Watermelon	92	200	62	1 slice watermelon
OTHER FOODS				
Bread, wholemeal	41	36	78	1 slice
Tomato soup, chilled	90	300	111	Half carton
Yogurt, fruit, low fat	78	150	135	Individual carton
Orange juice, freshly squeezed	88	150	50	Juice of 3 oranges

TOO MUCH OF A GOOD THING?

When considering phytonutrients, vitamins or minerals, it is important to recognise that if something found in a food has been proven to be beneficial, it does not necessarily follow that larger amounts of it, taken as supplements, are better. In fact, they sometimes can be harmful or have unexpected effects. Many of the recipes in this book use ingredients rich in phytonutrients so you and your baby can enjoy a good supply by selecting these healthy drinks.

times a day and can't keep any food or drink down, it is really important to go to the doctor as you can become dehydrated.

When you are breastfeeding, being adequately hydrated is important to ensure you have enough milk for your growing baby. Settling yourself down with a drink while you are feeding your baby is a good way of doing this. So have a look through the recipes for smoothies, juices and soups, which will provide additional nutrients as well as fluids.

DRINKS AS A SOURCE OF NUTRIENTS

Apart from your obvious need to remain well hydrated, drinks can provide useful amounts of key nutrients, at a time when you may not be able to manage whole meals. Often we think of drinks – a cup of tea or glass of water – in terms only of providing refreshment but by choosing carefully, it is possible to boost your nutritional intake of iron, calcium, vitamins B and C and even fibre.

Fruits and vegetables not only provide water (see table, page 11) and a range of different nutrients from beta-carotene to zinc, they also supply an enormous number of plant chemicals (phytonutrients), which scientists are only just beginning to understand. You may have heard about flavonoids found in tea and red wine, or lycopene in tomatoes. Most of these plant chemicals act as antioxidants, helping to inhibit harmful molecular reactions that can cause damage at cell level. It is thought this damage can lead to the development of chronic and ageing diseases such as cancers, heart disease, high blood pressure, rheumatoid arthritis and Alzheimer's disease.

For scientists it is a bit like discovering vitamins all over again, and it takes time to work out exactly what phytonutrients do in the body, how much of them we may need and how they react with one another and with vitamins and minerals. There is, as yet,

no research into their specific role in pregnancy, but as their role in reducing the risk of disease is becoming clear, it is reasonable to assume that they are helpful, not harmful, in pregnancy when taken in normal foods and drinks (see box, left).

If you have wisely chosen to reduce or cut out caffeine, tea, coffee, energy and cola drinks and chocolate will be off limits (see also page 18). By not drinking (or eating) them you'll be doing you and your baby a favour but you'll be doing yourselves a greater favour in improving your diet by replacing them with one of the drinks from the book. Your regular morning cappuccino or latte supplied essential calcium, protein and B vitamins from milk so you could swap to a dairy-based smoothie for breakfast, or drink it later in the day if you really can't face anything first thing.

You may also be thinking about cutting down on fizzy drinks; many of these simply supply calories from sugar and you'd be much better off with fresh home-made juices. These will supply more vitamins and phytonutrients than even fortified drinks can.

DRINKS TO HELP WITH PREGNANCY COMPLAINTS

Some women sail through pregnancy with a smile and not a whiff of nausea and others spend weeks feeling sick; some are anaemic, so take iron tablets; others become constipated and need laxatives; while still others suffer from heartburn and insomnia and wouldn't describe their pregnancy as enjoyable at all! Eating well, which includes what you drink, can help alleviate and even prevent some of these pregnancy ailments.

Several of the recipes in this book contain ingredients which are known for their positive impact on particular pregnancy symptoms (whether through scientifically conducted trials or long-term traditional use).

Nausea: It is thought that 50–75% of women experience some sickness and vomiting in pregnancy especially in the first trimester. Several factors can trigger this including the smell of food, cigarette smoke or perfume. For many women, drinks containing ginger help alleviate the symptoms and there are several in the book – Ginger and lemongrass cordial (page 114), which you could sip before getting out of bed, Fresh ginger and pineapple juice for breakfast (page 86) or Banana, pineapple and ginger smoothie (page 49) to keep nausea at bay during other times of the day. If your pregnancy includes the winter months, you could try Hot ginger and apple punch (see page 99), too.

Food aversions and cravings: Many women find they suddenly have an aversion to foods they previously loved or crave different foods or, rarely, non foods (a condition known as pica). This is perfectly normal and a result of hormonal changes. One of the most common cravings is for dairy foods so the many dairy-based smoothies and milky drinks in the book will help and provide you with essential nutrients such as calcium and riboflavin. Some women go off tea, coffee and alcohol very early in pregnancy and some speculate that this is nature's way of telling us to avoid these things. Replacing these drinks with healthy alternatives is important to ensure adequate hydration.

Constipation: Hormonal changes may trigger constipation, but the most common time for this preventable complaint is at the end of pregnancy when the rapidly increasing size of your baby can squash your intestines and slow everything down. Some women also find that iron tablets prescribed for anaemia predispose them to constipation. Preventing the condition is the best route, and this means ensuring that you are drinking at least the recommended 2.3 litres of fluids a day. Enjoy having drinks such as home-made smoothies and juices, or make a few simple soups which are nutrient rich and slip down easily when your stomach seems to have disappeared under the weight of the baby. High-fibre foods such as dates and prunes, beans and lentils also help, and these are found in several of the recipes, including Billion beans and garlic soup (page 57), Lentil and vegetable soup (page 61), Date and almond smoothie (page 47) and Spicy prune and apple smoothie (page 41). Avoid the need

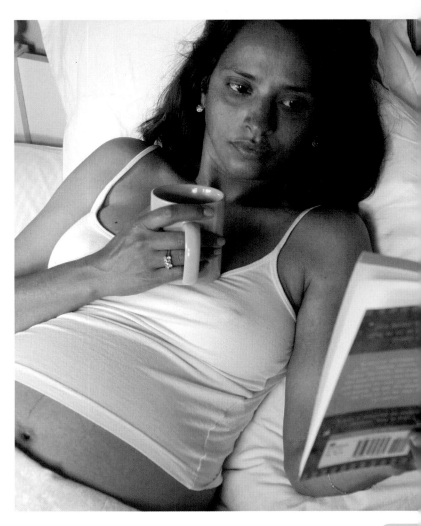

IF YOU HAVE GESTATIONAL DIABETES...

You should avoid the cordials in the book and limit the amount of fruit juice you drink to one 200 ml glass a day.

for iron tablets by having iron-rich soups such as Pea and spinach (page 54) and Lamb and pomegranate (page 75), which can also provide fibre and essential fluids. And try to stay active – moving around really does help to reduce the risk of constipation.

Anaemia: Anaemia occurs when you don't have sufficient iron in the diet and your body's stores are low. You are at risk if your pre-pregnancy diet was low in iron-rich foods, especially red meat. Common symptoms of anaemia are feeling breathless, faint and tired, and it is important to know that both mothers and babies can suffer. A baby gets less oxygen than he or she needs and this may slow down growth. You can find iron-rich recipes on pages 120–123.

Insomnia: Around three quarters of women experience sleep disturbance in pregnancy, especially in the last trimester when it can be difficult to get comfortable in bed. A milky drink such as Spiced milk (page 103)

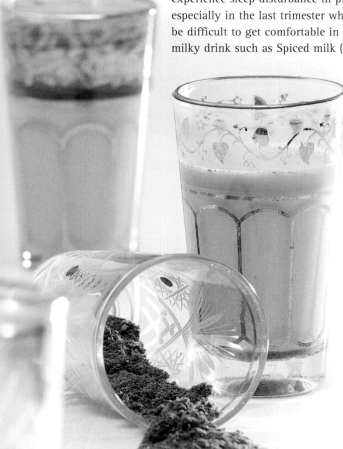

or home-made Chilli chocolate (page 104) can often help get you off to sleep. Some women find chamomile tea helpful and a flask of this by the bedside may be all you need to drift off to sleep.

Gestational diabetes: Around 2% of women suffer from gestational diabetes (that is, diabetes that comes on in pregnancy), mostly in the last trimester. If you are diagnosed with gestational diabetes, you will have additional tests and appointments to monitor your blood glucose levels and assess the growth of your baby. The condition can lead to a greater risk of complications for you and your baby so it is important to ensure you eat healthily and keep active. Your doctor or midwife is likely to suggest that you eat regular meals and snacks which contain high levels of slowly digested carbohydrate (that is, they have a low glycaemic index, or GI) and avoid excessive weight gain. Although they have not been specifically tested for GI values, the soups and dairy smoothies in this book are likely to be low GI, and make healthy snacks.

Heartburn: This uncomfortable burning sensation after eating is caused by the acid from the stomach coming back up your oesophagus. It is often worse in later pregnancy when the space for your organs becomes restricted due to the increasing size of your baby. It can be exacerbated by eating spicy or fatty foods, and by lying down soon after eating. Herbalists recommend drinking fennel tea, and you can also try mint teas, which are also good for the digestion (see page 106). To aid digestion, you could also drink the Spiced mint lassi (page 52) or add a few puréed mint leaves to the Watercress soup (page 67) or Pea and spinach soup (page 54). In late pregnancy, smaller meals such as soups may be preferable.

What not to drink

ALCOHOL IN PREGNANCY

Alcohol from your bloodstream passes through the placenta to your baby, where his or her liver needs to break it down. Your baby's liver, however, is not mature enough to do this effectively until you are at least halfway through your pregnancy.

Many studies have looked at the effect of alcohol on babies and it is clear that heavy drinkers are more likely to have babies who suffer from foetal alcohol spectrum disorder (FASD). The symptoms of FASD are low birth weight, facial deformities and lifelong disabling features such as learning difficulties and psychiatric problems.

Other research has focussed on the impact of binge drinking – that is, having more than 7.5 units of alcohol on a single occasion. Babies born to binge drinkers tend to be born prematurely and of low birth weight, and there is a higher incidence of miscarriage and still birth than in women who don't drink alcohol.

Studies, which look at light drinking in pregnancy – that is, having one or two units of alcohol once or twice a week, have produced conflicting results, and this is where controversy arises. What is known is that in the first trimester there is more likelihood of damage to a baby's organs, and some, but not all, studies have found an association between miscarriage and alcohol consumption in the first three months.

The long-term effects of drinking alcohol in pregnancy have been tracked in several large-scale studies. In two such studies, each examinining more than 11,000 children, the children of women who drank one or two drinks a week during pregnancy were no more likely to have behavioural difficulties or cognitive problems than those whose mothers didn't drink any alcohol at all. In fact, at age five, the children whose mothers were light drinkers were shown to have fewer behavioural problems and score higher on cognitive tests than the children whose mothers abstained completely in pregnancy. That said, even light drinking in pregnancy cannot be guaranteed to be risk free.

THE OFFICIAL LINE

In 2007, the UK Department of Health made it clear that pregnant women should not drink alcohol, but if they choose to do so, they should not drink more than one or two units once or twice a week. Pregnant women are advised not to get drunk or binge drink.

BREASTFEEDING AND ALCOHOL

The UK Royal College of Midwives advises women to avoid alcohol while breastfeeding, but other groups, such as the Breastfeeding Network, state that it is safe to drink in moderation. So what are the facts you need to help with your decision-making?

- Alcohol passes into your breast milk reaching a peak between 30–90 minutes after drinking.
- If you feed your baby during this time, he or she will certainly take in alcohol. This may make your baby agitated or could sedate him or her; some babies refuse to feed as the milk tastes different.
- If you plan to have an alcoholic drink, keep it to 1–2 units just occasionally, having fed your baby first, and avoid feeding for at least 2–3 hours after you drink.
- It is thought that the let-down reflex may be inhibited by alcohol.
- Alcohol is not stored in your milk; in time it clears from your body (and milk) so there is no need to express and tip any milk away.
- After drinking alcohol, do not go to sleep with your baby in your bed, or on a sofa or chair.
- Bear in mind that alcohol is a depressant. If you are feeling down, chat to your health visitor or doctor.

ALCOHOL UNITS IN COMMON DRINKS

Drink and strength (alcohol by volume, ABV)	Amount	Units of alcohol
White wine 13%	Standard glass 175 ml	2.3
White wine 13%	Large glass 250 ml	3.3
White wine 11%	Standard glass 175 ml	1.9
White wine 11%	Large glass 250 ml	2.8
Champagne 12%	Standard glass 175 ml	2.1
Champagne 12%	Large glass 250 ml	3.0
Red wine 14%	Standard glass 175 ml	2.5
Red wine 14%	Large glass 250 ml	3.5
Red wine 12%	Standard glass 175 ml	2.1
Red wine 12%	Large glass 250 ml	3.0
Rosé wine 10%	Standard glass 175 ml	1.8
Rosé wine 10%	Large glass 250 ml	2.5
Spirit (gin/ vodka) 37.5%	Single shot 25 ml	0.9
Spirit (gin/ vodka) 37.5%	Large single shot 35 ml	1.3
Spirit (gin/ vodka) 37.5%	Double shot 50 ml	1.9
Alcopop 4%	700 ml (70 cl) bottle	2.8
Alcopop 4%	275 ml bottle	1.1
Alcopop 5%	700 ml (70 cl) bottle	3.5
Alcopop 5%	275ml bottle	1.4
Cider 4.5%	440 ml can	2.0
Cider 7.5%	275 ml bottle	2.1
Cider 7.5%	500 ml can	3.8
Lager 4%	330 ml bottle	1.3
Lager 4%	440 ml can	1.8
Lager 5%	440 ml can	2.2

In 2008, the National Institute for Clinical Excellence (NICE) provided the following guidelines:

- Pregnant women and those planning a pregnancy should avoid drinking alcohol in the first three months of pregnancy, if possible, because it may be associated with an increased risk of miscarriage.
- If women choose to drink alcohol during pregnancy, they should drink no more than one to two UK units once or twice a week. Although there is uncertainty regarding a safe level of alcohol consumption in pregnancy, at this low level, there is no evidence of harm to the unborn baby.
- Getting drunk or binge drinking during pregnancy (drinking more than 7.5 UK units on a single occasion) may be harmful to the unborn baby.

Weighing up all this evidence should help you choose whether or not you will drink at all in pregnancy, and one of the purposes of this book, is to make sure you'll be able to produce interesting and healthier alternatives to alcoholic drinks. The recipe section includes ideas for mocktails and party drinks you can enjoy whether you are planning a pregnancy, pregnant or breastfeeding (or not!).

WHAT IS A UNIT OF ALCOHOL?

The drinkaware website available at http://www.drinkaware.co.uk/tips-and-tools/drink-diary/ has a useful calculator where you can add in the specific types and amount of alcoholic drinks, but a rule of thumb guide is included on the left.

IF YOU WERE DRINKING BEFORE YOU REALISED YOU WERE PREGNANT

Although it is advisable to plan for pregnancy, it is not uncommon for women to become pregnant unexpectedly. If your pregnancy was unplanned and you drank alcohol, the best advice is to stop drinking as soon as you realise that you are pregnant, and talk to your doctor if you still have any concerns.

CAFFEINE IN PREGNANCY AND WHEN BREASTFEEDING

Going off coffee can be one of the early signs that you are pregnant, but even if you can still tolerate it, how much should you be drinking while you are expecting?

In 2008, the UK government advised women that if they were planning a pregnancy or were pregnant, they should keep their caffeine intake to no more than 200 mg a day as there is a risk, albeit small, of fetal growth restriction, that is your baby will have a smaller than average birthweight. Some studies link consuming high quantities of caffeine to miscarriage. Caffeine crosses the placenta to your baby who cannot process it because he or she lacks the necessary enzyme to metabolise it. However, researchers have discovered that we all metabolise caffeine at different rates, depending on both our genetics and the environment, so some women may pass less to their babies than others.

If you drink caffeinated drinks while breastfeeding, your baby will also have a dose of caffeine as it takes a few weeks for a baby to develop the capacity to metabolise caffeine fully. For a baby less than one month old, it takes around four days for the amount of caffeine to be reduced by half, and then another four days for this to be halved again, and so on. However, by the time a baby is six months old, he or she can metabolise caffeine quite quickly – it takes just two and a half hours for the caffeine content to be halved, and the same to be halved again, and so on.

WHAT CONTAINS CAFFEINE?

When you are considering your caffeine intake, it's important to bear in mind that in addition to tea, coffee and cola, caffeine is also found in other beverages and some foods and over-the-counter medications, such as cold and flu remedies.

According to an EU code of practice energy drinks which contain more than 150 mg of caffeine per litre must carry a label declaring their caffeine content. They should carry a statement warning that they are 'not suitable for children, pregnant women and persons sensitive to caffeine'. As you can see from the table below, this amount of caffeine is often less than in a cup of coffee, but it is important that you are aware of the amount in a range of beverages.

Chocolate and cocoa contain small quantities of caffeine, the key being the darker the chocolate the higher the amount

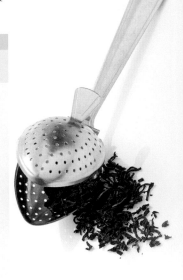

CAFFEINE CONTENT OF COMMON DRINKS

Type of drink	Quantity (approx)	Estimated amount of caffeine (mg)	Source
Instant coffee	One mug (260 ml)	100	*
	One cup (190 ml)	75	*
Black tea, infusion	One mug (260 ml)	50–75	*
	One cup (190 ml)	33–50	*
Drinking chocolate	Per pack instructions 200 ml	1.1–8.2	*
Filter coffee	Small (225 ml)	160	+
	Medium (350 ml)	240	+
	Large (450 ml)	320	+
Cappuccino or latte	Small (225 ml)	75	+
	Medium (350 ml)	75	+
	Large (450 ml)	150	+
Mocha	Small (225 ml)	90	+
	Medium (350 ml)	95	+
	Large (450 ml)	175	+
Flat white	Small (225 ml)	150	+
Americano	Small (225 ml)	75	+
	Medium (350 ml)	150	+
	Large (450 ml)	225	+
Energy drink (Red Bull)	473 ml can	151	Calculated from label
Cola drinks	330 ml can	11–70	*
70% cocoa dark chocolate	40 g	6	@
Milk chocolate	40 g	3	@
Cocoa powder	One cup (190 ml)	<1	@

* FSA Survey of Caffeine Levels in Hot Beverages, Food Information Sheet 53/04 April 2004, and FSA 2008
+ Starbucks nutritional information accessed March 2011
@ Green and Black's Organic Chocolate accessed March 2011

of caffeine, though in real terms it is not significant unless you are eating several bars of chocolate each day!

The table on page 17 shows the average amount of caffeine in a range of different drinks and foods. As you'll know from the coffee shops you visit, the strength of the brew is also determined by the barista. In the UK, the Food Standards Agency Food Surveillance Unit has measured caffeine levels in beverages, both brewed domestically as well as in the laboratory, and, not surprisingly, there are differences. The range of measurements is shown in the table. Also included are data from named sources in the UK.

ALTERNATIVES TO CAFFEINATED DRINKS

Keeping under the recommended 200 mg of caffeine per day need not be difficult – particularly as this book contains hot and cold beverages for every occasion – and being hydrated is more important than worrying if you have an occasional cappuccino. If you enjoy drinking tea, you can still have three or four cups a day, or choose decaffeinated versions. However, you may find that you are more willing to try new drinks and enjoy the book's caffeine-free herbal teas, or home-made smoothies and juices which will also provide you with additional nutrients.

Herbal or fruit teas or tisanes are now very popular and you may already enjoy some. These 'teas' are best defined as any infusion made from dried flowers, leaves or roots, which don't come from the tea plant *Camellia sinensis*. Mint tea, for example, is made from the leaves, chamomile the flowers and ginger the root of the respective plants. Many are a mixture of several different herbs or fruits. Drinking a few cups of these commercially available teas in pregnancy is perfectly safe for you and your baby. There is a concern, however,

> ## TAKING CARE OF YOUR TEETH
>
> During pregnancy, you need to pay attention to your dental hygiene. Visiting your dentist is free in pregnancy and until your baby is 12 months old. To look after your teeth:
>
> - Limit the amount of sugary acidic drinks you have and restrict these to meal times. Don't brush your teeth for at least an hour after having an acidic drink.
> - Drink plain water, herbal teas and dairy-rich drinks such as hot or cold milk in between meals.
> - If you need to sweeten a drink use a tooth-friendly sweetener (see box, page 108).
> - Brush your teeth at least twice a day with a fluoride-rich toothpaste.
> - If you need a drink in the night, have an unsweetened milky drink or water or herb tea. Your saliva production decreases at night so your teeth are more liable to plaque attack.
> - If you are vomiting a lot, your teeth are at risk of acid erosion, so ask your dentist for advice.

that certain herbal teas, particularly those that are drunk regularly in large quantities, may be unsafe due to their powerful medicinal effects. So avoid dong quai and black or blue cohosh during the entire nine months and raspberry leaf tea during the first three. There are safe home-made herbal teas that can help to alleviate common pregnancy complaints (see pages 106–107).

If you have cut out your usual drinks, it is wise to think carefully about what you are going to replace them with. If avoiding coffee and tea means you're tempted to increase the amount of fizzy drinks such as cola or lemonade, even if they are diet versions, think again. These sorts of drinks contain no pregnancy essentials – such as vitamin C, beta-carotene, calcium or fibre, which you and your baby need – and can be bad for your teeth (see box, right). Replacing every caffeinated drink with a juice isn't ideal either, as although you'll be getting plenty of vitamin C, it is easy to take in extra calories and sugars and you may gain weight more quickly than you should. So if you previously drank four cups of coffee a day, you should think about a range of replacements. Variety and moderation are key principles in good nutrition, pregnant or not. If you enjoy herbal and fruit teas continue to do so, but try different types, as well as fruit juices, water and milk-based drinks. For example, choose a milk-based drink to provide calcium and riboflavin, a juice or smoothie for a breakfast boost of vitamin C, and plain water to stay hydrated.

A significant issue with some drinks, especially carbonated drinks, fruit teas and some juices, is that they are very acidic. This acid can erode your tooth enamel allowing minerals such as calcium to leach out. In time, this weakens your teeth and leads to sensitivity, discolouration and other more severe consequences. To reduce the effect of acid erosion you should avoid swishing drinks around your mouth, and ideally drink acidic drinks through a straw. Although it seems counterintuitive, you can make the damage to your tooth enamel worse by brushing your teeth immediately after drinking an acidic drink.

Calcium and phosphorus, which are found in dairy products such as milk and yogurt, can help protect your tooth enamel. It is also known that casein, a protein found in milk, coats the enamel with a thin film, which helps protect teeth when exposed to acids in the mouth. So if you are going to have a smoothie in between meals, choosing one that is dairy based rather than 100% fruit means you will be protected against fruit acids by casein, calcium and phosphorus.

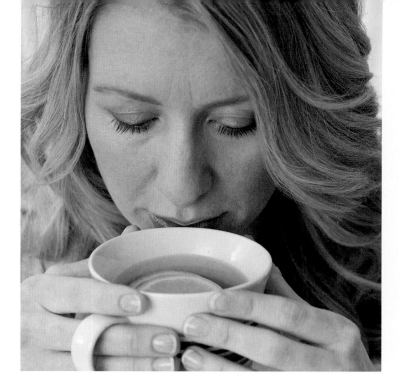

SUGARY AND ACIDIC DRINKS

Fruit juices and smoothies contain sugars, and these act on your teeth in the same way as the white sugar you may add to tea and coffee. Although they contain sugars, they do provide you with essential vitamin C, protective phytonutrients and a range of other vitamins and minerals which are important in pregnancy. A juice or smoothie is a much better alternative to a glass of squash or can of cola. However you need to be aware that the sugars contribute calories, and can also lead to tooth decay, so these drinks are best kept to meal times. Each of the recipes in this book has been nutritionally analysed using dietary analysis software so you will have an indication of how many calories and carbohydrates (sugars) each serving contains.

Sweeteners are safe in pregnancy, so if you prefer sweetened drinks, use one of the many types of sweeteners instead of table sugar. They won't decrease your liking for sweetened drinks, but at least your teeth will be better off.

Focus on pregnancy nutrition

The best time to think about eating well in pregnancy is before you conceive, but if your pregnancy, like many women's, is unplanned, what would have been ideal is no longer an option. It is, however, never too late to put healthy lifestyle modifications into practice, so instead of fretting about what can't be changed, change what you can now.

This section will provide you with information about some dietary essentials – in particular, the vitamins and minerals readily supplied by fruits and vegetables, which are significant ingredients in this book. The information is based on the latest research data, enabling you to make healthy choices of drinks as you plan to have a baby, as well as when you're pregnant or breastfeeding.

ESSENTIAL NUTRIENTS

The pages that follow flag up the significant nutrients needed for good health, as well as any recommendations for pregnancy and breastfeeding. *The Complete Pregnancy Cookbook* (Carroll and Brown, 2008) provides suitable dietary sources for these nutrients: this book is solely concerned with the nutrients found in drinks.

ENERGY – CALORIES

It comes as a surprise to many that the amount of energy (calories) you need when pregnant does not really increase until the last trimester. So it is not a case of having carte blanche to eat for two for nine months, and if you do so, you will gain additional weight you'll find hard to lose again. You only need an additional 200 calories in the last three months, because your body becomes very efficient at using energy and nutrients from stored tissue.

One source of calories is carbohydrates. These are usually starches and sugars. Most drinks, even those made from fresh ingredients, contain a high proportion of sugars, The way the body handles these sugars is not very different from the way it handles table sugars, so beware of adding extra weight through drinking too many juices and smoothies, and pay attention to dental hygiene too (see box, page 18). However, these fresh ingredients also contain a myriad of other dietary essentials

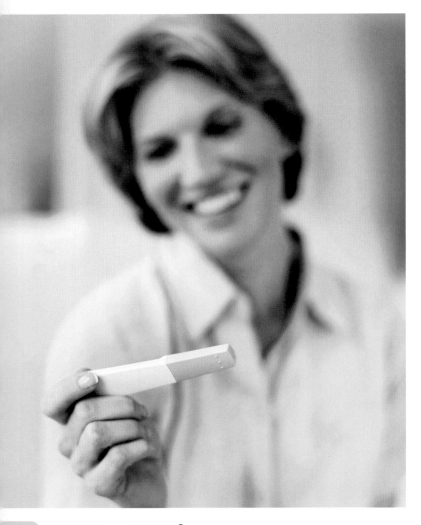

which pure white sugar doesn't, and these can make a significant contribution to your pregnancy diet.

If you are overweight or obese at the start of pregnancy, you need to take special care with what you eat, so that you don't gain weight too quickly. Rapid weight gain may increase your risk of pre-eclampsia and developing gestational diabetes. It is important, for example, to limit your consumption of fruit juices and avoid squashes and cordials. To help you choose wisely, every recipe has its calorie and carbohydrate (sugars) content listed. However, even if you are very overweight when you start pregnancy, it is not a good idea to try to lose weight now. It is important to ask your midwife or doctor for help in choosing foods wisely.

Breastfeeding is energy intensive, so additional calories are important to enable you to produce enough milk. This is the time when smoothies, soups and other energy-rich drinks can be really helpful as your fluid and energy requirements are high. Making batches of soups during pregnancy, and freezing them in portions for one or two people can be a great help at this time, as breastfeeding a baby can be very tiring and you may not have much time or inclination to be in the kitchen.

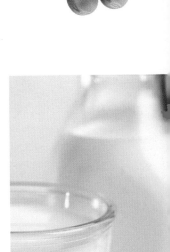

PROTEIN

Found in all your body cells, protein is needed for the growth of your baby. Most women in the UK consume more than enough protein so easily meet their pregnancy and breastfeeding needs.

FIBRE

In pregnancy it is especially important to keep things moving through your digestive system. An advantage of soluble fibre – found in oranges, apples and pears, as well as beans, peas and lentils and some cereal grains – is that it helps you feel fuller for longer, which can be useful if you are tempted to snack unhealthily. Insoluble fibre, found in fruits and vegetables – and wholegrain cereals – helps prevent constipation by keeping waste moving through the gut.

Smoothies contain a little dietary fibre because the whole fruit is puréed but juices which are pressed out of the fruit contain very little. This is the reason smoothies count as two portions of fruit and vegetables (of your recommended five a day) and juices as only one.

CALCIUM

Although calcium is essential for the proper growth and development of your baby's bones and teeth (your baby's first and adult teeth are present at birth!) as well as a healthy heart, muscles and nervous system, your calcium needs in pregnancy don't increase. Your pre-pregnancy diet, however, does have an effect on the calcium stores in your bones. If you start pregnancy with low amounts, you are more likely to be calcium deficient, which in turn raises your risk of pre-eclampsia. In the last trimester, your baby lays down a lot of bone and if you don't have adequate calcium from drinks (and foods), he or she will take it from your bones, leaving you with a greater risk of osteoporosis in later life.

Calcium requirements increase considerably for breastfeeding mums.

The good news is that it is not difficult to get enough calcium in the diet as milk and dairy products are excellent sources. Strict vegetarians and women who are intolerant of dairy products need to be especially careful, as although calcium is found in

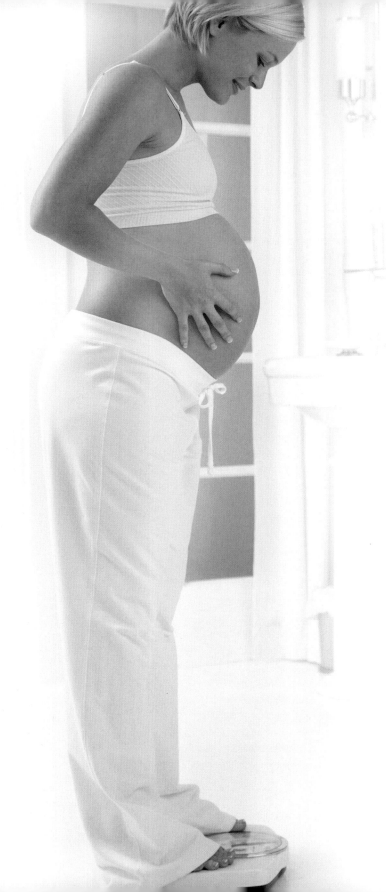

dark green leafy vegetables, almonds and tofu, the body tends to absorb it best from dairy products. Using calcium-enriched soya drinks instead of milk will help, but do seek professional advice about appropriate supplements if you think your intake is low.

Calcium works in conjunction with vitamin D, and a supplement may be recommended in pregnancy as few foods supply it and you can't always rely on sunshine to generate enough of your own.

The book contains a good selection of dairy-based recipes and most of those, which contain cows' milk or yogurt, can be made with a calcium-fortified soya alternative.

PHOSPHORUS

This bone-building nutrient is little discussed, largely as a deficiency is unlikely because it is found in many foods, particularly those that are rich in protein. Your needs don't increase during pregnancy, but almost double when breastfeeding so ensure you are eating a healthy balanced diet to obtain plenty of phosphorus.

POTASSIUM AND SODIUM

Both of these minerals are essential for health and are found in all body cells and fluids including blood and lymph. Having the correct balance of fluids, particularly in your blood, is crucial to your health. However, excess sodium (salt) increases your blood pressure, which is a risk factor for circulatory problems generally and hypertension in pregnancy.

If you start your pregnancy with high blood pressure, you need to be careful not to increase the amount of sodium (salt) you have in your diet. One way of helping control your blood pressure is to increase the amount of potassium you eat. Many fruits and vegetables are potassium-rich, so many of the juices and soups found in the book will help supply your needs.

Only the soup recipes in this book use salt and then a minimal amount. Where commercially made stocks are included, they are more dilute than recommended on the pack. If you have time, making your own stocks is a great idea (see pages 76–77).

MAGNESIUM

This mineral plays a huge number of roles in your body, pregnant or not. It assists with making protein and DNA for cells and tissues, the correct functioning of the nervous system and bone formation. It is also involved in regulating glucose and insulin metabolism, ensuring your blood sugar levels are kept constant. Your diet should contain plenty of magnesium as all of these functions affect your health and therefore that of your growing baby. Like calcium, magnesium is stored in your bones, so if your pre-pregnancy diet was poor, you will start to deplete your stores. There is also some evidence that low levels of magnesium are linked to leg cramps and pre-eclampsia.

In the UK, magnesium recommendations don't rise until you are breastfeeding, but it is worth eating magnesium-rich seeds, nuts and green leafy vegetables, and drinking milk, once you have conceived. Nibbling some seeds or nuts alongside a drink is a good way to maintain your levels.

IRON

Essential for the manufacture of blood cells needed for the rapid increase in blood volume during pregnancy and for placental growth, iron supplementation is not generally advised in the UK for women who eat a nutritious diet. However, many women go into pregnancy with low iron stores, especially if the pregnancy is unplanned, or they've had a baby within the last eighteen months and/or don't eat red meat or other iron-rich foods. The likelihood of low iron stores increases even more if you are still a teenager. Having low iron stores increases your risk of developing iron deficiency anaemia, and although your baby's need for iron will take precedence over your own, there is more chance he or she will be born underweight.

Developing iron deficiency anaemia in early pregnancy increases your risk of having a smaller placenta, which may influence the size of your baby. Becoming anaemic in your second trimester can increase your risk of giving birth prematurely and therefore of having a low birthweight baby. Recent studies have also found that there is a link between iron deficiency anaemia in the last trimester of pregnancy and schizophrenia in later life.

Your breast milk supplies iron to your baby and your ability to absorb iron from food improves after pregnancy. In the UK, there is no additional requirement for iron for breastfeeding mums.

Very few of these drinks recipes in the book actually contain sufficient iron to meet your needs. However, many of the

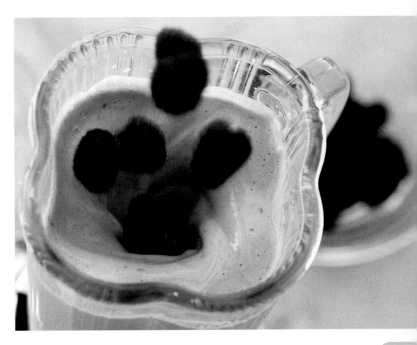

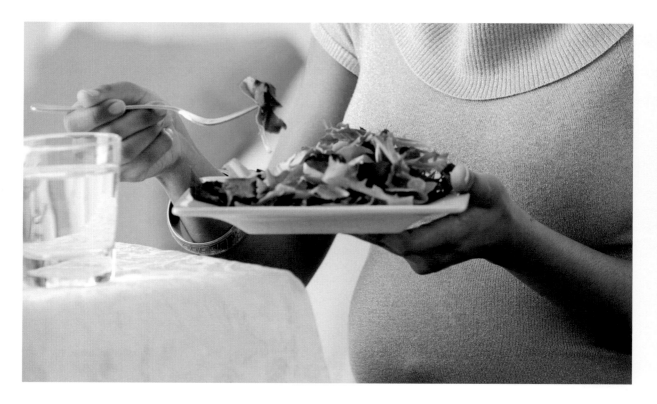

juices rich in vitamin C will increase your body's ability to absorb iron if you drink them when you eat high-protein foods.

VITAMIN A

Critical in pregnancy, vitamin A helps with the growth of all cells and is essential for the development of your baby's organs and circulatory, respiratory and nervous systems. It also helps boost your immune system so you can fight disease and infection, as well as maintain your vision and help the healthy development of your baby's eyes.

Vitamin A is a global term for retinol (found in animal foods) and carotenes (found in plant foods). The most commonly found carotene is beta-carotene which the body converts to retinol - six units of beta-carotene make one unit of retinol. In pregnancy, your need for vitamin A rises and there are many recipes in this book which can supply it.

Studies have shown the importance of eating well prior to pregnancy as it seems that low intakes of some micronutrients, including vitamin A, before you are pregnant not only influence your pregnancy but can also affect the quality of your breast milk.

RIBOFLAVIN

A B-group vitamin (B2), riboflavin has a role in energy release, and your requirements increase throughout pregnancy and when breastfeeding. If your diet doesn't contain sufficient riboflavin-rich foods when you are breastfeeding your milk will also be lacking in riboflavin. Dairy foods are a great source of this vitamin and many of the recipes provide this essential vitamin. A yogurt-based smoothie or hot milky drink when breastfeeding will help supply your needs.

If you don't eat dairy foods, consider enriched soya alternatives.

THIAMIN

Also known as vitamin B1 thiamin plays an important role in releasing energy from food. Your requirements only increase in the last trimester and when breastfeeding.

VITAMIN B6

Pyridoxine is a vitamin which can be depleted with the long-term use of the contraceptive pill. It is not readily stored in the body, so having a pregnancy diet rich in this nutrient is important. Your baby needs B6 for the normal development of his or her central nervous system and brain. It is also an important antioxidant, protecting against cellular damage and helping your immune defences. Many of the recipes in this book contain B6.

VITAMIN B12

This vitamin plays a crucial role in making red blood cells and genetic material, and is only found in algae or animal foods, meaning that strict vegetarians need to ensure a supply from a pregnancy supplement or fortified foods. Vitamin B12 (and folic acid) helps reduce levels of homocysteine, a potentially harmful substance which can increase your risk of circulatory and nervous system problems. It also increases the risk of birth defects, especially neural tube defects, premature birth and low birthweight. A good selection of drinks are rich in B12.

FOLATE

The synthetic form of folate, folic acid, is more usually known to women planning a pregnancy or newly pregnant. Folate is an essential nutrient as it is known to help reduce the risk of having a baby with neural tube defects (NTD). Taking a supplement of 400 micrograms a day from before conception to the twelfth week of pregnancy is essential, and for women who have already had a baby with an NTD this

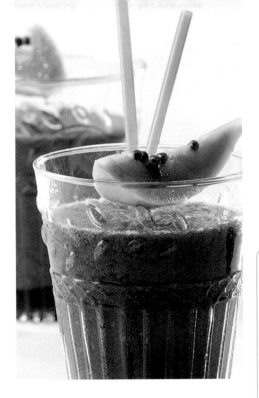

increases to 4 mg a day. It is known that low folate status in pregnancy can increase the risk of premature delivery.

Folates in foods are very susceptible to nutrient destruction, so it is important that food sources, of which the highest are vegetables, are carefully prepared and cooked to minimise losses.

VITAMIN C

Perhaps the best known of the antioxidant vitamins, vitamin C or ascorbic acid plays an important role in protecting cells against damage, keeping your immune system working correctly and ensuring the proper development and functioning of the placenta. Ascorbic acid helps the gut absorb iron from food, so it is an essential part of a pregnancy diet, especially as only tiny quantities can be stored in the body.

Vitamin C is found in many fruits and vegetables but can be destroyed by heating (see also pages 26–27). Most of the drinks in this book have been created to retain high quantities of vitamin C.

MAKE AND SERVE

Smoothies can be made with a range of different fruits as well as ice cream, sorbets and dairy ingredients such as yogurt or buttermilk. They should ideally be served straightaway to preserve their nutrient content, especially the water-soluble vitamins B and C, and folate, which decrease on storing.

Nutritional quality

THE FOOD INDUSTRY REGULATIONS

There are many books on juices and smoothies, some of which make extravagant claims about the vitamin or mineral content of the drinks, based on the inclusion of an ingredient in a recipe. So a vegetable juice containing a few spinach leaves may be said to be a good source of iron. In reality, the amount of iron provided by a few leaves would amount to a few micrograms, not even milligrams, so the juice is not exactly a good source.

The food industry has to comply with very stringent regulations on nutritional content before any sort of claims for its quality can be made on packaging. These are laid down in European Union law. Not many commercially available drinks or smoothies make any claims about their vitamin C, folate or any other micronutrient content. This is because nutrient losses in processing and storage can be great, so a food has to be an excellent source at the outset. Manufactured drinks are also often heat-treated to destroy bacteria which would shorten their shelf life and cause you harm, and these processes destroy some vitamins too.

The nutritional claims for recipes in this book are based on these food-manufacturing criteria. These strict regulations state that the food or drink must contain at least 15% of the recommended daily amount (RDA) of the nutrient to even mention that nutrient by name on the label. For example, if a manufacturer wants to claim that a drink is a 'source of' or that it 'contains' vitamin C, it must contain at least 9 mg of vitamin C per portion. For a claim that a food or drink is 'high in' or a 'rich source of' vitamin C, it must contain a minimum of 30% of the RDA, which is 18 mg. This is the amount that must be provided when you open the bottle or carton, not the amount contained in the original fruit prior to processing. Manufacturers therefore have also to take account of how much of any of these vitamins or minerals may be destroyed during any preparation or processing, which can be considerable.

PROCESSING LOSSES

The vitamins most liable to destruction are those which are water soluble – vitamin C, the B vitamins thiamin, riboflavin, niacin, B6 and B12 and folate. Different fruits and vegetables contain differing amounts of these vitamins, and the amount lost through peeling, cutting and chopping, through to puréeing varies, though these losses are not usually as great as losses through cooking. Perhaps not surprisingly, different methods of cooking using moist or dry heat affect the amount of vitamins lost, and often the longer the food is cooked, the

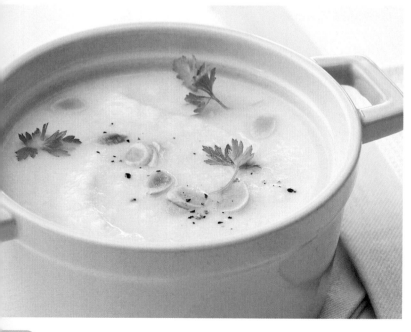

more vitamins are lost. One study which looked at the effect of cooking methods on the retention of folate (folic acid) found that 49% was lost when spinach was boiled compared to very little loss when steamed, but for potatoes boiling and steaming did not cause significant losses of folate. An Italian study showed that although the amount of vitamin C decreases considerably when vegetables are cooked, the amount of other important plant chemicals such as carotenoids and glucosinolates could increase. This underlines the importance of ensuring you have a good supply of different fruit and vegetables in your diet, which you eat both raw and cooked.

YOUR HOME-MADE DRINKS
There is little published research on vitamin losses when making smoothies and juices at home, but experts think that domestic puréeing should not lead to significant losses and the vitamin content should be very similar to the original fruit. The most likely losses occur through heat treatment and storage. Retail juices and smoothies may be pasteurised and chilled and these will cause some vitamin loss; long-life (ultra heat treated, UHT) beverages are likely to have significant losses because of the higher temperatures needed to destroy bacteria. Your home-made juices and smoothies, drunk when you make them, will therefore contain more vitamins than shop-bought varieties which have been subjected to heat treatment.

The majority of soups in this book are cooked, and nutrient losses through cooking have been taken into account. A research-guided estimate of 50% loss for vitamin C and folate has been used and 40% for other vitamins which are destroyed by heat. This means that for a soup to qualify for a claim

HIGH IN FOLATE	
Soups	**Juices**
Lamb and pomegranate page 75	Tomato, beetroot and celery page 93
Gazpacho page 63	Pomegranate and pineapple page 89
Pea and spinach page 54	Orange, grape and ginger page 81
Roasted roots page 69	Tomato, red pepper and carrot page 93

HIGH IN CALCIUM	
Smoothies & shakes	**Hot drinks**
Spiced mint lassi page 52	Chilli chocolate page 104
Chocolate surprise shake page 52	Spiced milk page 103
Date and almond smoothie page 42	Chai masala page 101
Mango lassi page 53	White chocolate and raspberry drink page 104

of 'source of' or 'high in', the basic ingredients have to be naturally high in that vitamin and after losing 40 or 50% through cooking, still have enough left to provide 15 or 30% of the RDA. If you look at shop-bought soups you'll see that none makes micronutrient claims. This is not just because it is expensive to carry out the laboratory analysis and even more expensive if claims are challenged by Trading Standards, but also because attaining these targets is difficult.

Your home-made soups are likely to contain the nutrients detailed if you use top-quality ingredients and follow the methods carefully. This will ensure you know that you and your baby are getting the best nutrition you can because you are in control.

Focus on ingredients

By making your own drinks, you can ensure a more nutritious, healthier drink than a supermarket equivalent as long as you choose your fruits and vegetables wisely.

SEASONALITY

Buying fruit and vegetables in season means that you are more likely to gain the optimum amount of vitamins from that food. In season means where you live; it may be summer somewhere else during your winter, but buying 'home-grown' seasonal fruit and vegetables helps local agriculture and cuts down on air miles.

However, even if you buy produce from your own country, its nutrient levels will not be consistent because growing conditions, season and time of harvest can affect the nutrient content. One study on broccoli, for example, demonstrated that it contained more vitamin C at the beginning of the harvest season compared to the end.

So although it is good to eat local produce in season, it is prudent to make sure that you know which fruits and vegetables contain key nutrients and when they are at their most abundant. In addition, many fruits and vegetables not grown in the UK can add variety and nutrients to your diet while you are pregnant and breastfeeding – particularly in winter – so use these to supplement your meals. These are not necessarily the exotics we associate with air miles such as mangoes, pineapples or papayas, as even lemons and limes are not commercially grown in the UK.

The table, right, shows the availability of fruit and vegetables in season in the UK month by month. It is important to note, however, that other UK-grown produce may still be available. These goods will have been harvested and stored under optimum conditions to prolong the 'season'. The table shows the season when produce is at its best.

THE BEST MONTHS FOR PRODUCE

January
rhubarb; beetroot, broccoli, Brussels sprouts, cabbages, carrots, celery, cauliflower, kale, leeks, parsnips, turnips

February
rhubarb; broccoli, Brussels sprouts, cabbages, carrots, cauliflower, kale, leeks, parsnips

March
rhubarb; broccoli, cabbages, carrots, cauliflower, kale

April
rhubarb; broccoli, carrots, cauliflower, cucumber, kale, lettuces, radish

May
rhubarb; cucumber, lettuces, radish, rocket, spinach

June
redcurrants, rhubarb, strawberries beetroot, broad beans, carrots, cauliflower, courgettes, cucumber, fennel, lettuces, peas, potatoes, radish, rocket, spinach, spring onions, turnips, watercress

July
cooking apples, blackcurrants, cherries, gooseberries, loganberries, raspberries, redcurrants, rhubarb, strawberries green and broad beans, beetroot, broccoli, savoy cabbage, carrots, cauliflower, celery, courgette, cucumber, fennel, lettuces, onions, peas, new potatoes, spinach, spring onions, tomatoes, turnips, radish, rocket, watercress

August
cooking apples, early-season eating apples, cherries, loganberries, plums, raspberries, strawberries

beans (all), broccoli, cabbage, carrots,
cauliflower, celeriac, celery,
cucumber, fennel, lettuces,
marrow, onions, parsnips, peas,
new potatoes, spring onions,
radish, rocket, spinach,
sweetcorn, tomatoes, turnips,
watercress

September
cooking apples, mid-season eating apples,
blackberries, pears, plums, raspberries, rhubarb
green beans, cabbages, cauliflower, celeriac, celery,
courgettes, cucumber, fennel, kale, leeks, lettuces,
marrow, onions, parsnips, maincrop potatoes, radish,
rocket, spinach, spring onions, squash, sweetcorn,
turnips

October
late-season eating apples, blackberries, pears, plums
runner beans, beetroot, broccoli, cabbages, carrots,
cauliflower, celeriac, celery, cucumber, fennel, kale,
lettuces, leek, marrow, parsnips, potatoes, pumpkin,
radish, spinach, spring onions, squash, swede,
sweetcorn, turnips

November
broccoli, cabbages, carrots, cauliflower, celeriac,
kale, leeks, parsnips, maincrop potatoes, pumpkin,
spinach, squash, swede, sweetcorn, turnips

December
broccoli, Brussels sprouts,
cabbages, carrots,
cauliflower, celeriac,
kale, leeks,
maincrop potatoes,
turnips

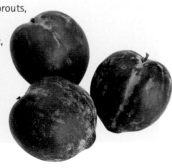

OTHER FACTORS INFLUENCING NUTRITIONAL CONTENT

Among the factors which can impact on the
nutritional value of the produce you eat are:

- The ripeness at harvest. Fully ripe
  tomatoes, for example, contain more
  lycopene (an antioxidant) than those
  which are not.
- Whether or not there is any physical
  damage such as bruising, or insect or
  disease damage. (This does not include a
  less-than-perfect appearance such as a
  mis-shapen tomato or pepper.)
- The nutrient content of the soil in which
  it is grown; this has more of an impact
  on minerals than vitamins. Selenium and
  iodine are elements which are particularly
  affected by the soil.
- How it is stored and/or processed at the
  packer and/or retailer; some fruits need
  to be chilled while others are better at
  room temperature, and vitamin content –
  especially vitamin C – declines in storage.
- How you store the product at home (see
  page 29).
- If cooking, the method you choose (see
  pages 26–27).

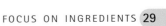

CHOOSING FRUIT AND VEGETABLES

There are several basic rules to consider when selecting fruits and vegetables. These are:

1 How the produce is being displayed – is it chilled, sitting in the sun, loose, wrapped or bagged? How long may it have been there?

2 On bagged or labelled produce choose the latest use-by date you can find, which may be at the back of the shelf.

3 Look for bruises or other blemishes; these may indicate the produce has been badly handled or had an infestation or disease.

4 Particular advice applies to specific fruit and vegetables. The table on the right offers a brief summary of what you should look for.

SHOULD I CHOOSE ORGANIC?

The decision to buy organic food is often based on the assumption that it is healthier than conventionally produced food. However its perceived nutritional superiority has not been confirmed despite many conflicting studies over the years. The most comprehensive recent review conducted independently for the UK Food Standards Agency showed that there were no significant differences in the vitamin or mineral content of organic and conventionally grown fruit and vegetables.

However there are other reasons why you may choose to eat organic foods, including environmental concerns and the possible effect of pesticide residues, which are potentially harmful. Most governments have stringent rules on permissible levels, and fruit and vegetables are regularly tested to ascertain whether or not there are harmful pesticide residues, which could be transferred to your baby in utero, or in breast milk. Most countries carry out dietary surveys on a regular basis and test all the components of the diet to monitor whether there are residues of pesticides, herbicides and fungicides.

It is known that organochloride pesticide residues accumulate in fatty tissues and this means that they can be stored in breast tissue and so may be passed to the baby when you are breastfeeding. However these particular pesticides, as well as polychlorinated biphenyls and dioxins, have been banned in many countries, markedly diminishing the risk to you and your baby. It is important to note that the benefits of breastfeeding far outweigh the minuscule danger posed by potentially harmful residues.

WHAT TO LOOK FOR

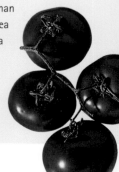

Berries and cherries
These should have a bright clean skin, and no evidence of mould. Select firm dry fruit and don't buy punnets with signs of juice as fruits are likely to be mushy.

Grapes
When you pick up a bunch of grapes, none should fall off. They should have a bloom and be firm.

Mangoes
Mangoes should give slightly when pressed but not be squashy. Smell the stem end for a delicious aroma which is apparent when fruits are ripe.

Melons
Lightly press the opposite end to the stem, which should yield slightly to show it is ripe. A watermelon which resonates when tapped is ripe and will be juicy.

Papaya
Handle a papaya with care. It should feel heavy for its size and have a blemish-free skin. Gently squeezing a ripe fruit will leave an impression.

Peaches, nectarines and plums
Skins should be blemish-free, fruits should yield slightly when gently pressed and have a delicious aroma. Plums may have a bloom.

Pears
Usually picked under-ripe, pears can be ripened at home in a paper bag at room temperature. Some varieties are harder than others, but generally the area near the stalk should yield a little when it is ripe.

Pineapple
The leaf crown should be glossy so you can pluck out

a leaf with a little tug, indicating it is ripe. Check the skin for blemishes, and only buy if the skin is firm and the fruit smells sweet.

Pomegranates
Look for a smooth glossy skin and check that the fruit feels heavy for its size.

Bagged leaf salads
Check the bag is intact. These should have a long sell-by date and no browning or wilted leaves.

Cauliflower
Beware those which have no leaves as this may indicate they are older and the leaves have softened so have been removed. Check that it smells fresh and that the 'curds' are white and spot free.

Celery, cucumber, beans, fennel and rhubarb
Stalks should be firm to the touch, and stiff so you could break them rather than bend if you were to try.

Leaves such as spinach, chard, rocket, watercress, and herbs
Leaves should be crisp with a freshly cut stem. Avoid slimy or broken leaves.

Peppers of any colour
Peppers should feel firm and heavy, and have glossy skins. The stalk should look fresh and not withered.

Root vegetables such as carrots, beetroot, parsnips and potatoes
Brush off any soil and check the skin has not been pierced by insect holes, and is not damaged or mouldy. Potatoes should have no eyes or green colouration.

Tomatoes
Look for a blemish-free smooth skin. These can be ripened at room temperature for a few days.

STORING FRUIT AND VEGETABLES
In an ideal world, you would buy fruit and vegetables in season at least twice a week to ensure they were at their freshest. However, most of us do our shopping once a week, just topping up when necessary and also buy frozen produce which tends to be just as nutritious as fresh. Some produce needs storing in the fridge; others may need to be left at room temperature to ripen or just taste their best; still others are frozen and need to stay that way until you want them. Here are a few tips about what to store where and for how long.

First of all, it's worth noting that some fruit naturally produces ethylene, a harmless gas which causes ripening in other fruits and vegetables. This can be helpful if you want to ripen something faster – for example, pop a banana in a bag with peaches or an avocado to speed up their ripening. However, they can go off faster once they are ripe, so pop them in a plastic bag away from other produce.

Most produce should not be washed before storing as this will hasten its deterioration, but placing in a plastic bag in the fridge will keep it fresher for longer. Some products, for example mushrooms, are best kept in a paper bag.

If you are going to use fruit such as apples, pears, citrus fruit and already ripe mangoes, pineapple and pomegranates within a couple of days, you can keep them on the worktop. If they are for later in the week, pop them in the fridge in a plastic bag.

Root vegetables such as carrots, potatoes and parsnips, and squashes and pumpkins, as well as onions and garlic, can be kept in a cool dark place, or if you have space, the fridge is fine.

Salad leaves, herbs and vegetables such as beans, mangetout, broccoli, peppers and ripe tomatoes should be kept in the crisper drawer, preferably in a plastic bag, or they will keep longer in a fridge bag.

Drink-making equipment

When you are considering buying equipment it is a good idea to think through carefully what you intend to use it for, and whether it has more than one use. For example, you may fancy a smoothie maker to produce your own delicious pregnancy drinks, but a blender or food processor can do this too and be used for puréeing your baby's food when you start weaning. Once you've decided what you want, use these guidelines to help you choose a particular model.

GENERAL FACTORS TO CONSIDER

1 How easy is it to clean, which parts – if any – can go in the dishwasher?
2 How easy is it to assemble?
3 What quantity of food can it take – is this enough if you were to make a dish for four or six?; will it process tiny quantities of food as well?
4 Does it come with a sealed or spill-proof lid to prevent liquids spurting out of the lid?
5 How powerful is the motor – measured in watts – and is this sufficient for your needs?
6 Does the instruction manual give you ideas and recipes?

SMOOTHIE MAKERS

These are specialised blenders some of which have a tap so your drink comes out of the bottom (rather than your having to dismantle the jug). They are designed so that the ingredients, whether fruits, ice cream or yogurts, are directed towards the blades to be blended quickly. The motor size influences the speed and efficiency of the smoothie maker, and the larger the motor the noisier they tend to be. Consider how many speed settings you want and whether a pulse setting is useful. Check

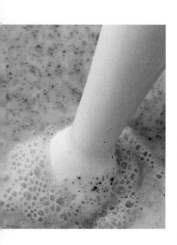

whether a model can also process ice cubes if you like your smoothies very cold. Some models have a central insert in the lid so you can add ingredients while the motor is running. If you are making smoothies for yourself alone a small (1 litre) jug may be ample, but if you are looking to the future when you are encouraging your child to eat fruit and vegetables a larger or family-size (2 litre) model may be more appropriate.

JUICERS

There are many ways to extract juice from fruit and vegetables. For citrus fruit, a simple reamer, or citrus press, in which your muscles supply the energy is the cheapest option. However, if you want to juice a lot of citrus fruits an electric citrus press may be the answer. Other juice extractors, which are ideal for a wide range of fruit and vegetables, have their limitations for citrus fruit unless they have a special citrus attachment. If they don't, then before juicing you have to remove the peel and pith from the fruit as these tend to be bitter.

Most electric juicers on the market in the UK are based on a centrifugal extraction system. Here the fruit or vegetables are fed through a funnel and come into contact with a wire mesh basket and high-speed rotating blades. The juice passes through the mesh and into a jug or through a spout straight into your glass. If you don't like the froth which accompanies the juice, some machines have a separator panel in the collecting jug.

You may want to consider the size of the funnel as some will take whole fruit such as apples, while others require you to chop the fruit before juicing. As with a smoothie maker, think about the power of the motor and the number of speed settings.

Preparing produce for juicing

Many fruits do not need peeling but all should be washed thoroughly before juicing. Fruits with stones such as cherries, plums and peaches should have these removed. Some fruits, such as bananas and avocadoes, are not suitable for juicing, and are better puréed in a blender or processor. Apples and pears, which make delicious juices, brown very quickly so you may want to stir in a little lemon juice or a sprinkling of vitamin C powder (available from health-food stores, chemists and on line) to discourage this.

Vegetables are delicious juiced, so choose those which are crisp and firm such as carrots, beetroot, celery or cucumber. It is easier to feed leaves such as spinach and watercress in with other ingredients.

Drink the juices straightaway for maximum nutrient content, adding ice if you wish.

BLENDERS

There are two basic types of blenders: free-standing models have a jug which tops the motor and look not dissimilar to a smoothie maker, and the more portable hand or stick blender which you place straight into the food. Some have attachments that enable you to purée small quantities of food which can be helpful for making baby foods or grinding spices. Hand blenders are ideal for making soups as they can be placed straight into a saucepan, and some have wider heads to do this without splashing.

For making smoothies, a free-standing model is ideal but some of the hand blenders have attachments including ice-crushing blades which will enable you to quickly make a smoothie for one.

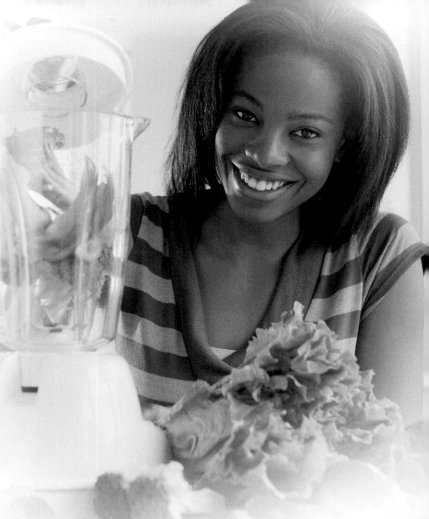

FOOD PROCESSORS

Food processors carry out more functions than blenders or smoothie makers, and many have attachments to enable you to chop, mix, whisk, slice, shred, blend and even grind foods, as well as extract juice with a citrus press. Prices usually reflect the type of motor, the cheaper models having a series motor with individual power settings, and the more costly an induction motor which automatically adjusts the power to suit the food being processed.

Consider the type of functions you want to use your processor for, and if you are only going to make smoothies, or blend soups, you probably don't need a processor.

CAUTION

Some food processors can spurt liquid when processing, which can be dangerous if you are blending a hot soup.

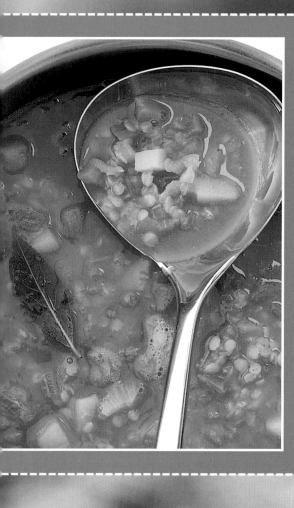

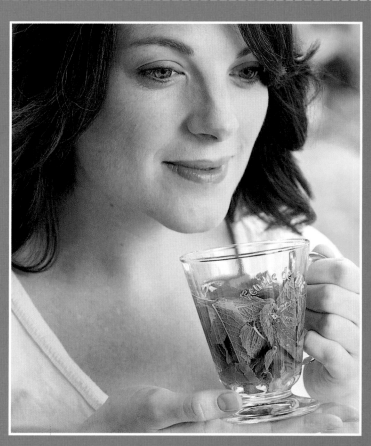

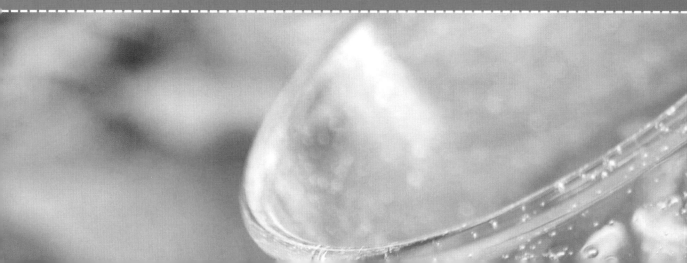

RECIPES

Enjoy the bounty of the seasons, whether from your garden, the supermarket shelves, farmers' markets or farm shops, and create nutrient-rich drinks that will nourish you and your growing baby. As well as tasting delicious, you'll have the satisfaction of knowing that you are making drinks filled with essential vitamins and minerals to help both of you at this special time.

Each recipe offers a range of nutritional information, including a calorie count (kcal) and carbohydrate content (including sugars) in grams (g) per serving, when made according to the recipe instructions. In addition, the smoothies, soups and hot drinks give a protein and fat (including saturates) content in grams (g). Protein and fat contents of the other drinks are negligible or 0 g. A full nutritional breakdown of all recipes is given on pages 120–123.

SMOOTHIES & SHAKES • SOUPS • JUICES • PARTY DRINKS
HOT DRINKS • CORDIALS & COLD DRINKS

SMOOTHIES & SHAKES

FIVE A DAY

Smoothies officially count as two portions of your five a day. This is because they include the whole fruit and not just the juice. You also benefit from having the fibre, which would be lost in juice making.

MANGO AND PASSION FRUIT SMOOTHIE

For those hot days or when you don't feel like eating, this delicious smoothie will give you a boost of energy along with a huge supply of carotenes and vitamin C.

Good for: Boosting energy
High in: Vitamin C, carotenes
Source of: Fibre

Makes 1 310 ml serving
141 kcal • 1.7 g protein
32.7 g carbohydrate (of which 29.6 g sugars)
0.5 g fat (of which 0.3 g saturates)

½ large mango (150 g prepared weight), cut into cubes (see below)
2 small scoops passion fruit sorbet (about 50 g)
Juice of ½ lime (10 ml)

1 Place the mango in the blender and whizz until smooth.
2 Add the passion fruit sorbet and lime juice and blend again briefly.
3 Pour into a glass and serve straightaway.

• *Not suitable for storing.*

HOW TO PREPARE A MANGO

Mangoes can be a bit tricky to prepare as there is a large central stone to which the fibrous flesh often sticks. When using in drinks, either cut into slices or cubes. Use a sharp knife to work lengthways along the fruit in line with the shape.

SLICING A MANGO
1 Use a sharp knife to remove the peel.
2 Hold the fruit firmly, starting with the flat 'face' of the flesh in the palm of your hand.
3 Cut off long, slim wedge-shaped slices. Some of the slices near the narrow side of the stone will be misshapen.

CUTTING A MANGO INTO CUBES
1 Slice the fruit lengthways on either side of the flat stone, cutting as close to the stone as possible but without piercing it.
2 On your two stoneless 'cheek' sections, slice the flesh in a lattice pattern, cutting down to the peel but not piercing it.
3 Push the peel inside out with your thumbs. Then use the knife to cut away cubes.

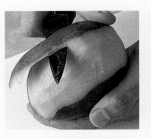
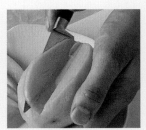
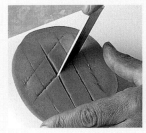
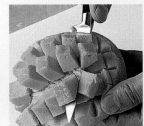

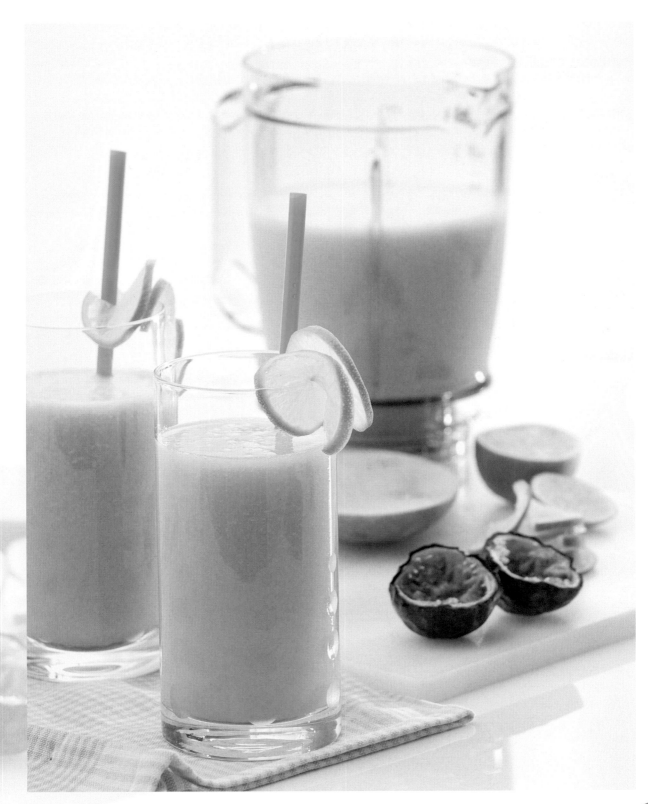

MANGO, APRICOT AND PINEAPPLE SMOOTHIE

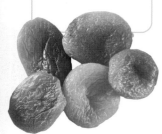

BUYING DRIED FRUIT

Dried fruit such as apricots, prunes and raisins provide useful amounts of iron. Vitamin C, found in many fruits, helps the body absorb iron which is essential in preventing anaemia and helping your baby's blood and tissue development.

The dried apricots in this smoothie provide a small but useful amount of iron, which is easily absorbed thanks to the vitamin C content; the fibre in the apricots is useful for relieving constipation. If you're making fresh pineapple juice, you'll need a juicer for this recipe.

Good for: Preventing anaemia, relieving constipation
High in: Vitamin C, fibre
Source of: Iron

Makes 1 280 ml serving
163 kcal • 2.4 g protein
37.1 g carbohydrate (of which 36.8 g sugars)
0.5 g fat (of which 0 g satuates)

100 ml pineapple juice, preferably freshly made
½ medium mango (120 g prepared weight), cut into cubes (see page 36)
3–4 ready-to-eat dried apricots (30 g)

1 Place the pineapple juice, mango cubes and apricots in a blender and process until smooth.
2 Serve straightaway.

• *Vitamin C content will be lost on chilling though this smoothie can be stored in the fridge in a covered glass for a few hours.*

MANGO AND PEACH SMOOTHIE

MANGOES

The mango originated in southeast Asia and is today grown in many parts of the world; they are available year round in the UK.

Pick mangoes that are plump and heavy for their size, and which are fragrant. Mangoes are ripe when you can indent them slightly with your thumb.

Peaches and and their smoother-skinned cousins, nectarines, finish their season as mangoes start, so you can have a cheap and nutritious summer smoothie, which is full of carotenes your body converts into essential vitamin A.

Good for: Boosting immunity
High in: Vitamin C
Source of: Carotenes

Makes 2 310 ml servings
Per serving 130 kcal • 1.6 g protein
30 g carbohydrate (of which 29.6 g sugars)
0.4 g fat (of which 0 g saturates)

175 ml unsweetened apple juice
1 medium mango (250 g), cut into cubes (see page 00)
2 medium ripe peaches or nectarines (285 g), peeled, quartered and stones removed

1 Place apple juice, mango cubes and peaches or nectarines in a blender and process until smooth.
2 Serve straightaway.

• *Not suitable for storing.*

TROPICAL DELIGHT SMOOTHIE

This mixture of fruits makes a smoothie with all the taste sensations of an exotic island. Put a few ice cubes in the blender to chill it down on a hot day or use frozen fruit instead of fresh for the same effect.

Good for: Quenching thirst
Source of: Vitamin C

Makes 2 275 ml servings
Per serving 104 kcal • 1.4 g protein
23.4 g carbohydrate (of which 22.4 g sugars)
0.5 g fat (of which 0.2 g saturates)

*100 ml unsweetened pineapple juice, preferably
    freshly made*
150 ml coconut water
*½ small melon (160 g), such as Honeydew or
    Galia, cut into chunks*
1 medium banana (100 g), cut into chunks
Ice cubes (omit if using frozen fruit)

1 Place all the ingredients in a blender and
   process until smooth.
2 Serve straightaway.

• *Not suitable for storing.*

COCONUT 'WATER'

Coconut 'water' is the liquid which comes
from fresh or green coconuts. As these are
often not readily available unless you happen
to live in the tropics, you can use pre-packed
coconut 'water', which is available in
supermarkets. Coconut 'milk' – not to be
confused with coconut 'water' – is made from
the shredded flesh of the coconut mixed with
water while coconut 'cream', also made from
the flesh is much thicker.

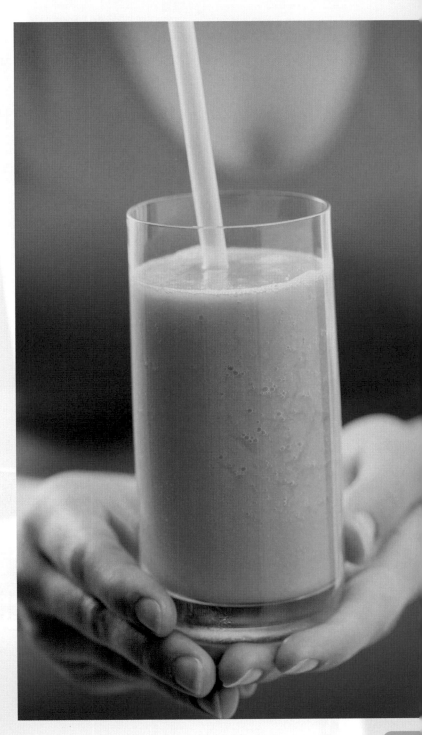

NECTARINE, RASPBERRY AND ORANGE SMOOTHIE

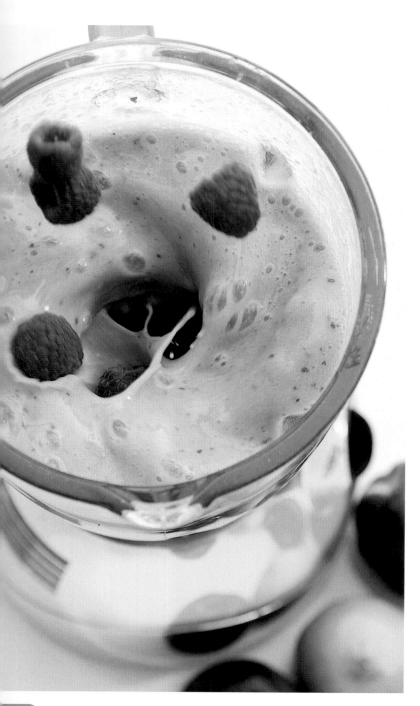

This combination of summer fruits provides a big vitamin C boost. Raspberries contain iron too: not enough to make an iron-rich claim, but enough to help your increased needs during pregnancy.

Good for: Boosting immunity, quenching thirst
High in: Vitamin C
Source of: Folate

Makes 1 360 ml serving
113 kcal • 3.7 g protein
23.8 g carbohydrate (of which 23.8 g sugars)
0.4 g fat (of which 0 g saturates)

100 ml orange juice, preferably freshly squeezed
75 g fresh or frozen raspberries
1 medium nectarine (150 g), quartered and stone removed

1 Place all the ingredients in a blender and process until smooth.
2 Serve straightaway.

• *Not suitable for storing.*

RASPBERRIES

The leaves of the raspberry plant can be made into an infusion which is said to make labour easier. Eating the raspberry fruit itself during pregnancy is safe but raspberry leaf infusions should only be drunk in the last few weeks of pregnancy (see page 107).

VANILLA, BANANA AND PRUNE SMOOTHIE

This is breakfast in a glass, especially if you use full-fat Greek yogurt. Both the banana and the prunes are good sources of potassium, a vital pregnancy mineral, so make this smoothie a regular feature of your pregnancy diet.

Good for: Preventing constipation
Source of: Fibre, calcium, riboflavin

Makes 1 285 ml serving
318 kcal • 10.1 g protein
34 g carbohydrate (of which 32 g sugars)
15.7 g fat (of which 10.3 g saturates)

150 g Greek yogurt, reduced-fat if preferred
1 small banana (80 g)
3–4 ready-to-eat prunes (30 g)
1–2 drops vanilla extract

1 Place all the ingredients in a blender and process until smooth and creamy.
2 Pour into a glass and serve.

• *This smoothie will keep in the fridge in an airtight container for 24 hours.*

VANILLA

The seed pod of a species of orchid, vanilla is used principally for its sweet flavour rather than any nutritional benefits it may offer. It makes a great addition to banana recipes like this smoothie.

SPICY PRUNE AND APPLE SMOOTHIE

Constipation is a common pregnancy complaint and you can prevent it by having plenty of fibre, and plenty of fluids. This smoothie provides both. For a tangy flavour, choose an apple variety such as Granny Smith, or, for a sweeter taste, Red Delicious.

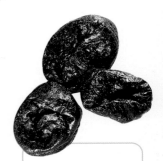

Good for: Preventing constipation
High in: Fibre
Source of: Calcium

Makes 1 355 ml serving
238 kcal • 7 g protein
49 g carbohydrate (of which 47.4 g sugars)
1.6 g fat (of which 0.8 g saturates)

1 large banana (120 g)
200 ml unsweetened apple juice
10–12 ready-to-eat prunes (120 g)
200 g low-fat natural yogurt
½ tsp mixed spice

1 Cut the banana into chunks and place in a blender.
2 Add the remaining ingredients and process until smooth.
3 Serve or store.

• *The smoothie is not particularly rich in vitamin C, so may be stored for up to 24 hours in an airtight container in the fridge.*

PRUNES

Prunes are a fantastic source of potassium, which helps maintain blood pressure at a healthy level. This is especially important during pregnancy to reduce the risk of pre-eclampsia.

CHERRY HEAVEN

Cherries aren't around for long, so make the most of the cherry harvest in summer by enjoying this heavenly smoothie. Its wonderful colour ensures a vibrant drink, full of protective plant substances and powerful antioxidants.

CHERRIES

These juicy, red fruits contain good levels of vitamin C and antioxidants, which help boost your immune system and encourage healthy tissue growth during pregnancy.

Cherries can be sweet or tart depending on their variety, so experiment until you find which you prefer. Both types contain phenolics, plant compounds that have anti-inflammatory effects, although tart varieties contain the most.

You can store cherries for a few days in the fridge, and they will keep frozen for up to a year without the taste being affected. You may prefer to stone them before freezing.

Good for: Boosting immunity
Source of: Calcium, riboflavin

Makes 1 275ml serving
178 kcal • 7.5 g protein
16.1 g carbohydrate (of which 16.1 g sugars)
9.3 g fat (of which 5.2 g saturates)

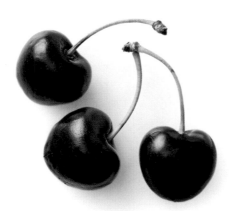

12–14 ripe cherries (100 g), washed and pitted
50 g blueberries
100 g Greek yogurt, low-fat if preferred

1 Place the cherries and blueberries in the blender and process until smooth.
2 Gently pulse in the yogurt, keeping the mixture fairly thick.
3 Serve straightaway.

• *Not suitable for storing.*

HOW TO STONE CHERRIES

You can use a paring knife to slice around the cherry stone, but this can result in losing a lot of the flesh. A cherry stoner, however, can make this tedious task much easier and preserve more of the fruit. You can use the same device for stoning olives too.

1 Remove the green stem from the cherry.
2 From the stem end, carefully use the plunger to push the stone out through the other end of the cherry.

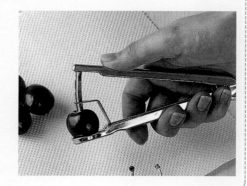

RASPBERRY, POMEGRANATE AND PAPAYA SMOOTHIE

This great smoothie is made up of three delicious and healthy fruits. Raspberries are full of protective antioxidants including vitamins C and E, quercetin, lutein and myricetin, which protect cells against damage. Freezing does not affect these substances and if you like your smoothie chilled, you can use raspberries straight from the freezer for this recipe. Pomegranates (see box, right), are rich in antioxidants while papayas are an excellent source of vitamin C. You'll need a juicer for this recipe to make the pomegranate juice.

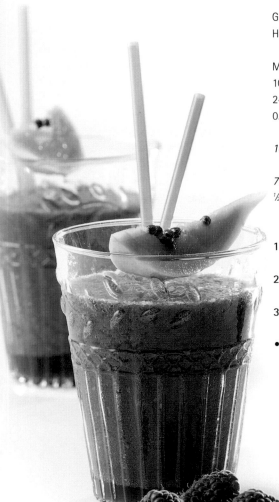

Good for: Boosting immunity
High in: Vitamin C, fibre

Makes 1 325 ml serving
108 kcal • 1.8 g protein
24.3 g carbohydrate (of which 24.3 g sugars)
0.3 g fat (of which 0 g saturates)

*100 ml freshly made pomegranate juice (from
   1 medium pomegranate)*
75 g raspberries, fresh or frozen
*½ medium ripe papaya (125 g), peeled, seeds
   removed and cut into chunks*

1 Pour the pomegranate juice into the
   blender.
2 Add the raspberries and papaya and blend
   until smooth.
3 Serve straightaway.

• *To retain vitamin C content, serve
   straightaway, though this smoothie can
   be stored in the fridge in a covered glass
   for a few hours.*

POMEGRANATES

Pomegranates' rich supply of antioxidants; vitamins A, B, C and E; folate, potassium and calcium makes them ideal during pregnancy, when these vitamins and minerals are essential for the healthy development of a baby. Select thin-skinned, heavy fruits, as half the pomegranate's weight is made up of edible seeds from which the juice comes.

NECTARINE AND PASSION FRUIT SMOOTHIE

This smoothie, which contains calcium and riboflavin from the yogurt, will go down easily on days when you are struggling to eat well. The natural sugars in the fruit will also give you a quick energy boost.

PASSION FRUIT

There are two main types of passion fruit, or granadilla: purple varieties are subtropical, and yellow varieties tropical. Purple ones are wrinkly rather than smooth when ripe. Choose fruit that is heavy for its size and firm. Passion fruits are high in beta-carotene, which the body converts into vitamin A, important for good fetal development and for strengthening the immune system.

Good for: Bone development
High in: Fibre
Source of: Calcium, vitamin C, riboflavin

Makes 1 400 ml serving
204 kcal • 8.5 g protein
39 g carbohydrate (of which 37.1 g sugars)
1.5 g fat (of which 0.8 g saturates)

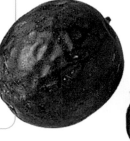
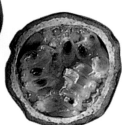

2 ripe passion fruit
1 nectarine or peach (150 g), peeled, stone removed, and quartered
1 small banana (80 g)
100 g low-fat natural yogurt

1 Cut the passion fruit in half and scoop the seeds into a small sieve. Press through and catch the juice for the recipe, and discard the seeds.
2 Place the passion fruit juice in a blender and add the nectarine or peach, banana and yogurt and process until smooth.
3 Serve straightaway.

• *Not suitable for storing.*

NATURAL YOGURT

Plain yogurt is easily digested and can sometimes be tolerated by people who are unable to digest lactose – the sugar found in milk – as the bacteria which make the yogurt also break down lactose. If you have a severe lactose intolerance, however, yogurt should be avoided. Plain yogurt is a great addition to any diet but is especially useful in pregnancy for times when it is difficult to eat.

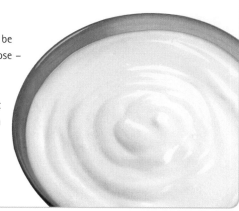

BERRY BOOST SMOOTHIE

In the summer there are many red and purple fruits to choose from and all provide a burst of phytochemicals, protective plant substances. Plenty of farms offer strawberry- and raspberry-picking, which is a great way to get the freshest fruit possible. If you're making this smoothie in winter, however, you can use frozen berries.

Good for: Aiding digestion
High in: Vitamin C
Source of: Fibre, calcium

Makes 1 275 ml serving
98 kcal • 5.8 g protein
16 g carbohydrate (of which 15.2 g sugars)
1.2 g fat (of which 0.7 g saturates)

8–10 medium, ripe strawberries (100 g), hulled
50 g blueberries or bilberries
100 g low-fat natural yogurt

1 Place the ingredients in a blender and process until smooth.
2 Serve straightaway.

• *Not suitable for storing.*

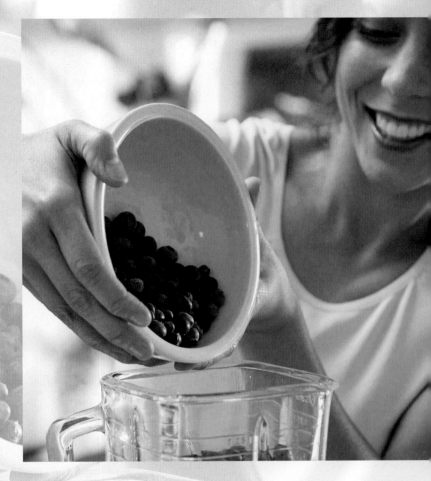

FRESH OR FROZEN?

Frozen fruits and vegetables can be just as nutritious as fresh. Frozen raspberries, blueberries and blackcurrants may lose some vitamin C when stored for up to one year in the freezer, but levels of other phytochemicals remain almost the same. However, frozen fruit can be much cheaper than fresh when out of season and when used in juices and smoothies the vitamin content will be considerably higher than shop-bought produce which will have beeen heat-treated before transporting.

An alternative to buying frozen fruit is to buy fresh – or pick your own – when it is in season and freeze it yourself. Rinse berries (except for blueberries, which are best washed before using), hull strawberries, and drain. Spread the berries in a single layer on a tray (to prevent them lumping together) and put them in the coldest part of your freezer overnight, so they become completely frozen.

It is best to use frozen fruit straight from the freezer for smoothies as this minimises any vitamin C loss in thawing.

GRAPEFRUIT

A good source of vitamin C and lycopene and a powerful antioxidant, grapefruit also contains fibre, folate, bioflavonoids, potassium, calcium and phosphorous – all of which are great in pregnancy. The bioflavonoids reduce water retention and swelling in the legs, and the fibre from the pith aids digestion.

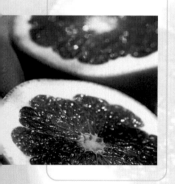

RED BREAKFAST SMOOTHIE

This vitamin C-rich smoothie is a wonderful way to start the day. Use the ripest, sweetest strawberries to complement the tartness of the grapefruit juice. You can use either pear or banana to thicken the mixture and add fibre.

Good for: Reducing water retention
High in: Vitamin C
Source of: Fibre

Makes 1 260 ml serving
(with pear) 77 kcal • 1.3 g protein
17.3 g carbohydrate (of which 17.3 g sugars)
0.2 g fat (of which 0 g saturates)
(with banana) 91 kcal • 1.6 g protein
20.4 g carbohydrate (of which 19.6 g sugars)
0.3 g fat (of which 0 g saturates)

½ ruby grapefruit (150 g)
8–10 medium, ripe strawberries (100 g), hulled
½ small pear (50–60 g) or ½ small banana (40 g), peeled and chopped

1 Squeeze the juice from the grapefruit, which should yield around 60–75 ml. Pour into the blender.
2 Hull the strawberries and add to the blender along with the pear or banana.
3 Process until smooth and serve straightaway.

SUMMER FRUITS SMOOTHIE

This delicious smoothie benefits from the antioxidants found in red and purple summer fruits; choose those you like the most and combine with a pear for fibre. On really hot days, add some ice cubes to the blender to chill it down.

Good for: Boosting folate
High in: Vitamin C, fibre
Source of: Folate

Makes 1 275ml serving
88 kcal • 1.6 g protein
19.4 g carbohydrate (of which 19.4 g sugars)
0.4 g fat (of which 0 g saturates)

50 ml unsweetened apple juice, freshly pressed if possible
75 g raspberries, or strawberries, cleaned and any stalks removed
25 g blackcurrants, stalks removed, or blueberries
1 small ripe pear (100 g), peeled, cored and cut into chunks

1 Place the prepared fruit in a blender, adding ice if you like a chilled drink.
2 Blend until smooth and pour into a serving glass.
3 Serve straightaway.

• *To retain vitamin C content, serve straightaway, though this smoothie can be stored in the fridge in a covered glass for a few hours.*

DATE AND ALMOND SMOOTHIE

Fortified dairy replacements such as fortified soya milk and yogurt are useful alternatives if you cannot tolerate dairy products, as they provide essential calcium and vitamin D. These nutrients are vital for the development of your baby's bones, teeth, heart and brain and, if you plan to breastfeed, the vitamin D can augment the proportion contained in breast milk.

Good for: Bone development
High in: Calcium, vitamin D
Source of: Fibre

Makes 1 275 ml serving
145 kcal • 7.6 g protein
19.7 g carbohydrate (of which 19.1 g sugars)
4 g fat (of which 0.7 g saturates)

50 g fresh dates, stones removed
100 ml fortified light soya milk
100 g fortified soya yogurt
2 drops almond extract

1 Place all the ingredients in a blender and process until smooth.
2 Serve in a glass.

• *This smoothie can be kept in the fridge in an airtight container for up to 24 hours.*

DATES

Naturally sweet, dates are rich in fibre, and contain potassium which helps control your blood pressure. They are also a source of folate, which is important in early pregnancy. Dates also help constipation, but should be eaten in moderation as they have a high sugar content.

KIWI, PEAR AND GRAPE SMOOTHIE

If you have a juicer, you can make fresh juice from green seedless grapes. However, you can use off-the-shelf unsweetened grape juice. If you buy white grape juice, you'll retain the lovely green colour of this smoothie. As you can't enjoy the antioxidant benefits of wine, enjoy the flavonoid-rich grapes in this smoothie instead.

Good for: Boosting immunity
High in: Vitamin C

Makes 1 350 ml serving
147 kcal • 2 g protein
33.1 g carbohydrate (of which 32.7 g sugars)
0 g fat

100 ml unsweetened white grape juice or
    30 green grapes (150 g), juiced
1 small ripe pear (100 g), peeled, quartered and
    pips removed
2 kiwi fruit, peeled

1 Place the grape juice, pear and kiwi in a blender and process until smooth.
2 Serve straightaway.

• *To retain vitamin C content, serve straightaway, though this can be stored in the fridge, covered, for a few hours.*

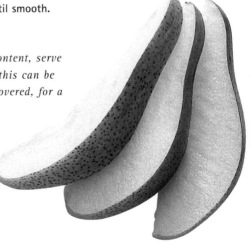

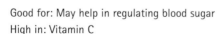

KIWI, APPLE AND
BANANA SMOOTHIE

Using a green apple such as a Granny Smith in this recipe not only provides a lovely tang, but a vibrant green colour, too. However, if you have a sweeter tooth, you should choose a Gala, Red Delicious or Rome. To get the most fibre out of this smoothie, juice your own apple; one large one (about 200 g) will be sufficient. If you use a ready-prepared apple juice, choose a cloudy one, or one from a variety such as English Cox, which also has a 'bite' to it.

KIWI FRUIT

The bright green flesh of the kiwi fruit is an excellent source of vitamin C, essential for a healthy immune system; two kiwi will supply your daily requirement in the last trimester. The potassium content helps to counteract the high sodium levels typical of a Western diet, helping to regulate your blood pressure.

Good for: Aiding digestion
High in: Vitamin C
Source of: Fibre

Makes 1 320 ml serving
178 kcal • 2.3 g protein
40.4 g carbohydrate (of which 38.1 g sugars)
0.9 g fat (of which 0 g saturates)

100 ml unsweetened apple juice, preferably freshly squeezed
2 kiwi fruit, peeled and quartered
1 medium banana (100 g), peeled

1 Place all the ingredients in a blender and process until smooth.
2 Serve straightaway.

• *Not suitable for storing.*

GRAPE, PINEAPPLE AND
BANANA SMOOTHIE

Grapes are naturally very sweet and their fructose (fruit sugar) content means they have a low glycaemic index (GI). Foods with a low GI help to regulate blood sugar levels, which is important during pregnancy. If you're making fresh pineapple juice, using a juicer will give a smoother consistency than if you use a blender.

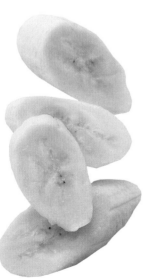

Good for: May help in regulating blood sugar
High in: Vitamin C

Makes 1 310 ml serving
179 kcal • 1.6 g protein
42.1 g carbohydrate (of which 40.5 g sugars)
0.4 g fat (of which 0 g saturates)

1 small banana (80 g)
18–20 seedless red grapes (100 g), washed and stalks removed
100 ml unsweetened pineapple juice, not from concentrate if possible, or 1 pineapple juiced

1 Peel the banana and break into chunks.
2 Place all the ingredients in a blender and process until smooth.
3 Serve straightaway.

• *Not suitable for storing.*

PINEAPPLE, BANANA AND GINGER SMOOTHIE

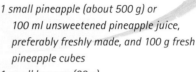

Ginger has long been used during pregnancy to alleviate nausea. This zingy smoothie may be just what you need when you don't feel much like eating but need some energy to keep going; it also can help kick-start your digestive system.

Good for: Combating nausea
High in: Vitamin C
Source of: Fibre

Makes 1 320 ml serving
161 kcal • 1.5 g protein
37.5 g carbohydrate (of which 35.6 g sugars)
0.6 g fat (of which 0 g saturates)

1 small pineapple (about 500 g) or
    100 ml unsweetened pineapple juice,
    preferably freshly made, and 100 g fresh
    pineapple cubes
1 small banana (80 g)
1 tsp lime juice
1 tsp fresh ginger root, grated

1 If using a whole pineapple, prepare as below and use approximately half the slices to make the juice and the other half to cut into cubes.
2 Place all the ingredients in a blender and process until smooth.
3 Serve straightaway.

• *To retain vitamin C content, serve straightaway, though can be stored in the fridge in a covered glass for a few hours.*

PREPARING A PINEAPPLES FOR JUICING

Using a juicer produces a smoother juice and enables you to extract juice from the nutrient-rich skin if the pineapple is organic. A ripe pineapple should smell sweet and yield slightly when the base is squeezed gently. Using a large knife, cut off the plume and the base of the pineapple. Carefully slice off the skin, dig out any remaining spikes or eyes using a small knife or the end of a potato peeler and slice around the hard core.

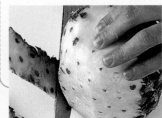
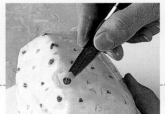

PAPAYA, GRAPE AND PEAR SMOOTHIE

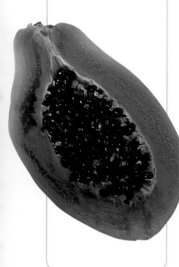

PAPAYA

Papayas are particularly rich in vitamin C but are not as acidic as other fruit. Avoid unripe, green-coloured papayas as in Asia these are reputed to cause miscarriage. Studies on rats have borne this out, but no studies have been carried out on humans.

Red wine is thought to improve cardiovascular health, probably due to resveratrol, a substance found in red grape skins that can lower cholesterol and prevent fats from sticking together and clogging the arteries. Drinking dark grape juice made with skins may be just as heart-healthy as drinking red wine, without the associated health hazards.

Good for: Boosting immunity
High in: Vitamin C
Source of: Carotenes, fibre

Makes 1 295 ml serving
106 kcal • 1 g protein
24.9 g carbohydrate (of which 24.9 g sugars)
0.3 g fat (of which 0 g saturates)

1 medium, ripe papaya (250 g), peeled, deseeded and cut into cubes
150 ml red grape juice, fresh or ready prepared
Juice of ½ lime (10 ml)
1 medium pear (150–160 g), peeled, quartered and pips removed

1 Place all the ingredients in a blender and process until smooth.
2 Serve straightaway.

• *Not suitable for storing.*

PAPAYA AND STRAWBERRY SMOOTHIE

As both papayas and strawberries are rich in vitamin C, carotenes and antioxidants, this breakfast smoothie provides a vitamin pick-up for the summer months when strawberries are at their peak. Strawberries are available in supermarkets from April to December, but the tastiest fruit is pick-your-own between June and mid-August.

Good for: Boosting immunity
High in: Vitamin C, carotenes
Source of: Fibre
Makes 1 340 ml serving
102 kcal • 1.8 g protein
23.1 g carbohydrate (of which 23.1 g sugars)
0.3 g fat (of which 0 g saturates)

100 ml freshly squeezed orange juice
Juice of ½ lime (10 ml)
½ medium ripe papaya (125 g), peeled, seeds removed and cut into chunks
6–8 medium-sized ripe strawberries (80 g), hulled

1 Place the cut papaya and lime juice in a blender and process until smooth.
2 Add the strawberries and orange juice and blend until smooth and thick.
3 Serve straightaway.

• *To retain vitamin C content, serve straightaway. However, because this smoothie is so high in vitamin C, it can be stored in the fridge in a covered glass for a few hours.*

STRAWBERRY MILKSHAKE

This traditional milkshake is made with fresh strawberries rather than strawberry syrup. Strawberries are an excellent source of vitamin C – this recipe alone will provide you with all the vitamin C you need when breastfeeding, a massive 100 mg a day. Milk is a great source of calcium, phosphorus and potassium. All of these are essential in pregnancy for the healthy development of you and your baby.

Good for: Bone development, tissue growth
High in: Vitamin C
Source of: Calcium, folate

Makes 1 285 ml serving
165 kcal • 5.8 g protein
23.3 g carbohydrate (of which 23.2 g sugars)
5.5 g fat (of which 3,4 g saturates)

8–10 medium, ripe strawberries, hulled (100 g)
100 ml semi-skimmed milk
60 g strawberry ice cream (about 1 scoop)

1 Place the strawberries a blender, pour in the milk and blend until smooth.
2 Add the ice cream and pulse until the mixture is just smooth.
3 Serve straightaway.

• *Not suitable for storing.*

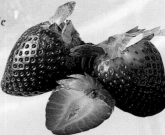

STRAWBERRIES

Juicy and full of vitamin C, strawberries also contain folate, calcium, iron, potassium and manganese – all vital pregnancy minerals. The berries also contain the protective plant nutrient, ellagic acid, also found in black tea. If you've been cutting back on tea because of its caffeine content, strawberries will top this up, too.

DAIRY-FREE STRAWBERRY MILKSHAKE

For those who are unable to tolerate both milk and soya products, shakes are a no-no. However, by using ingredients which are dairy and soya free, along with vitamin C-rich strawberries, shakes can be a delicious reality.

Good for: Boosting immunity
High in: Vitamin C
Source of: Fibre

Makes 1 310 ml serving
138 kcal • 1.2 g protein
30.3 g carbohydrate (of which 24.1 g sugars) •
1.3 g fat (of which 0 g saturates)

10–12 medium, ripe strawberries (120 g), hulled
100 ml rice milk
60 g dairy- and soya-free raspberry or strawberry sorbet or frozen dessert (about 1 scoop)

1 Place the strawberries in a blender and add the rice milk and sorbet.
2 Blend until smooth and serve straightaway.

• *Not suitable for storing.*

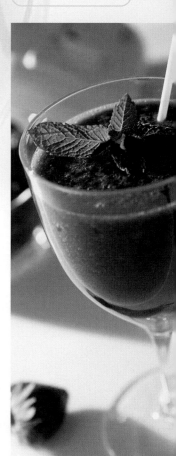

CHOCOLATE SURPRISE SHAKE

If you are a chocolate lover then you'll enjoy this shake, which has a secret ingredient: prunes. As it is based on milk, you'll also have a great supply of calcium, riboflavin and essential iodine, too. Share it with your partner for a delicious treat.

Good for: Bone development
High in: Calcium
Source of: Riboflavin, iodine

Makes 2 280 ml servings
Per serving 215 kcal • 7.9 g protein
29.1 g carbohydrate (of which 27.7 g sugars)
7.5 g fat (of which 3.9 g saturates)

300 ml semi-skimmed milk
5–6 ready-to-eat prunes (60 g)
125 g chocolate ice cream (about 2 scoops)

1 Place all the ingredients in a blender and process until smooth.
2 Serve straightaway.

• *Not suitable for storing.*

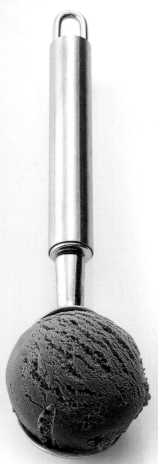

SPICED MINT LASSI

This simple traditional unsweetened lassi contains two digestive aids. The first is mint leaves – fresh or frozen – which are believed to help relieve heartburn and the second is cardamom, which has been used for centuries to improve digestion.

Good for: Relieving heartburn, aiding digestion, combating nausea
High in: Iodine, calcium

Makes 1 225ml serving
114 kcal • 9.6 g protein
14.3 g carbohydrate (of which 13.5 g sugars)
2 g fat (of which 1.4 g saturates)

200 g low-fat natural yogurt
1 cardamom pod, seeds removed and crushed
1 heaped tsp chopped mint leaves, fresh or frozen
Few ice cubes, optional
Few toasted cumin seeds, optional

1 Place the yogurt, crushed cardomom and mint in a blender.
2 Add ice cubes, if using, and blend.
3 Serve straightaway, topped, if desired, with a few freshly toasted cumin seeds.

• *Lassi is best served straightaway, but if you don't add ice cubes you can keep the drink for 24 hours in an airtight container or covered glass in the fridge.*

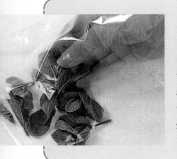
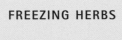

FREEZING HERBS

Herbs can be frozen in two ways: either pack them into labelled freezer bags or chop finely and half-fill ice cube trays, topping up with water. Herbs can be kept in the freezer for up to six months.

MANGO LASSI

Lassis originally come from India's Punjab region, and are yogurt-based drinks, which can be either savoury or sweet. This one uses cardamom, which has a delicate, spicy flavour that works well with mango, but its use is optional. Sprinkle with cinnamon for an added kick, if you prefer.

Good for: Bone development
High in: Calcium

Makes 2 250 ml servings
Per serving 128 kcal • 7.6 g protein
20.5 g carbohydrate (of which 19.9 g sugars)
1.7 g fat (of which 1.1 g saturates)

*½ large mango (150 g prepared weight), cut into
   cubes (see page 36)*
300 g low-fat natural yogurt
*1 cardamom pod, seeds removed and 1 or 2 finely
   crushed, optional*
Few ice cubes, optional
Lime zest

1 Place the mango in a blender with the
   yogurt and cardamom, if using.
2 Blend until smooth, adding a few ice cubes
   if you want a really cold drink.
3 Serve topped with a little lime zest.

• *Lassi is best served straightaway, but if
you don't add ice cubes you can keep the
drink for 24 hours in an airtight
container or covered glass in the fridge.*

CARDAMOM

In small amounts, cardamom may help relieve
nausea and morning sickness. The antioxidant
potential of cardamom is great but not
realised as generally
only tiny
quantities are
used.

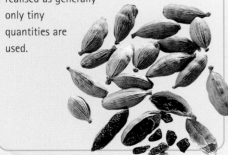

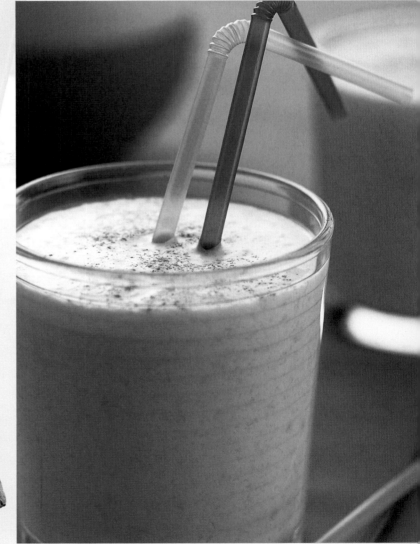

SOUPS

PEA AND SPINACH SOUP

An extremely quick and highly nutritious soup, pea and spinach will be among your favourites as soon as you try it. Vary it by adding mint or fresh coriander, or add a swirl of cream for a creamy twist. Finish with a few croûtons if you like.

WHY FROZEN MAY BE BEST

Frozen vegetables are frozen immediately after harvesting, which locks in their nutrient content. 'Fresh' vegetables in the supermarket, however, have often spent days in transit or storage and much of their goodness has been lost.

Good for: Preventing constipation
High in: Fibre, folate
Source of: Iron, vitamin C

Makes 4 350 g servings
Per serving 120 kcal • 8.4 g protein
12.2 g carbohydrate (of which 4.5 g sugars)
4.2 g fat (of which 0.5 g saturates)

1 tbsp vegetable oil
1 medium onion, chopped
450 g frozen peas
200 g frozen leaf spinach
750 ml vegetable stock (see page 75)
Black pepper
Nutmeg, freshly grated

1 Heat the oil in a non-stick saucepan and fry the onion gently until softened.
2 Add the frozen peas, spinach and stock and bring to the boil.
3 Simmer for 5 minutes until the peas are just tender
4 Blend until smooth, season with black pepper and nutmeg, and serve with a drizzle of single cream, if desired.

• *To retain vitamin C content, serve straightaway. However, this soup can be stored in the fridge in an airtight container for 24 hours, or may be frozen.*

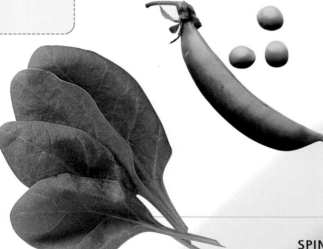

SPINACH

Spinach is a very nutrient-rich food, but once picked its nutritional value depreciates quickly. In some recipes, therefore, it's a good idea to choose frozen spinach over fresh or pre-packed (see box, left). Bursting with caretonoids and flavonoids, spinach is also high in vitamin C, manganese, selenium and zinc. Zinc is important for a baby's developing nervous system and bones as well as cell production and repair.

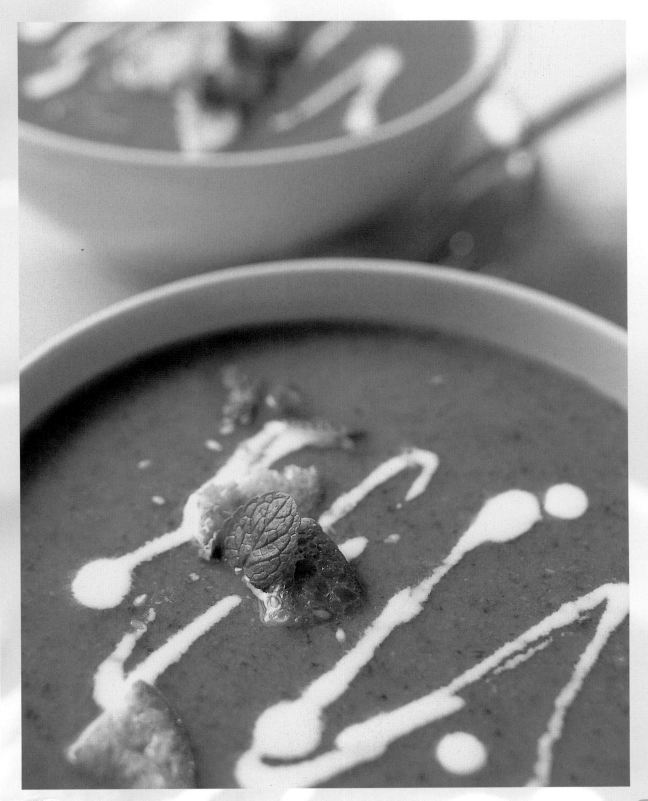

CREAMY GREEN PEPPER SOUP

This soup has a surprise ingredient which you won't taste but that will provide you with essential folate. So if you've read down the list of ingredients and identified your least favourite vegetable, rest assured that its presence won't make itself known.

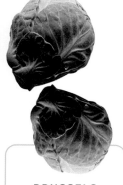

BRUSSELS SPROUTS

Though not to everyone's taste, Brussels sprouts are in fact a powerhouse of vitamins and minerals, notably vitamin C and folate. Folate is an essential nutrient, especially in early pregnancy, for preventing neural tube defects in a developing baby.

Good for: Boosting immunity
High in: Vitamin C
Source of: Fibre, folate, calcium

Makes 3 333 g servings
Per serving 193 kcal • 8.6 g protein
18.8 g carbohydrate (of which 14.6 g sugars)
9.3 g fat (of which 3.2 g saturates)

25 g sunflower or olive oil spread
1 large onion, finely chopped
2 medium green peppers, stalk and seeds removed, and roughly chopped
8–10 Brussels sprouts (140 g), trimmed and finely chopped
1 rounded tbsp plain flour
500 ml semi-skimmed milk
200 ml vegetable stock or water with 1 level tsp reduced-salt vegetable bouillon (see page 77)

1 Heat the spread in a non-stick saucepan and gently fry the onion for a few minutes until it becomes translucent.
2 Stir in the peppers, cover, and allow to sweat over a low heat for 10 minutes.
3 Now stir in the sprouts and flour, and gradually mix in the milk. As the mixture thickens, add the stock or water and bring to the boil, stirring constantly.
4 Cover and simmer for 10 minutes.
5 Blend until smooth and serve with garlicky croutons.

• *To retain vitamin C content, serve straightaway, though this soup can be stored in the fridge in an airtight container for 24 hours.*

PEPPERS

Peppers belong to the same family as chillies and there are many different varieties, each with a different colour and shape. The green bell pepper would ripen to red and taste sweeter if left on the plant, but in this creamy soup recipe its stronger flavour works well with milk. Yellow peppers are sweeter still.

BILLION BEANS AND GARLIC SOUP

This soup contains as many beans as you want it to: whether you buy a three- or ten-bean mix it is up to you. All contain roughly the same mix of beneficial nutrients including many of the vitamin B group, iron and lots of fibre. It's a good idea to make a bumper batch, and freeze some for other occasions when you may feel less like cooking.

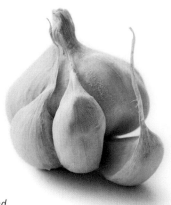

Good for: Preventing anaemia, preventing constipation
High in: Fibre, carotenes
Source of: Iron, thiamin

Makes 6 384 g servings
Per serving 268 kcal • 15.6 g protein
28 g carbohydrate (of which 4.6 g sugars)
10.3 g fat (of which 3.4 g saturates)

240 g lardons
1 medium onion, finely chopped
3 sticks celery, finely chopped
2 large carrots, finely diced
60 g pearl barley
4 cloves garlic, crushed
Few sprigs rosemary
3 bay leaves
200 g mixed dried beans, soaked overnight and boiled until soft, or 2 x 400 g cans of beans of your choice, drained
1.5 litres chicken or vegetable stock (see pages 76–77)
2 tbsp chopped parsley

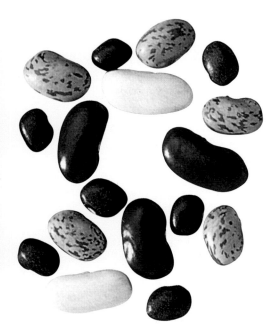

1 Place the lardons in a large saucepan and heat gently, stirring constantly to allow the fat to ooze out.
2 Add the onion, and cook for 4–5 minutes until just softening.
3 Stir in the celery, carrot and barley along with the garlic and herbs.
4 Add the beans, pour in the stock and bring to the boil.
5 Cover and simmer for 40–50 minutes until the vegetables and beans are all tender.
6 Sprinkle on the parsley and serve.

• *This soup keeps well for 48 hours in the fridge, but can be frozen in an airtight container for up to six months.*

THE BENEFITS OF BEANS

Beans are a low-fat, high-fibre food. In addition to providing magnesium and folate, they are also a good source of iron. A healthy intake of iron ensures a good supply of haemoglobin, the component of the blood responsible for transporting oxygen around the body, and ensuring you have the energy you need to cope with the demands of pregnancy. Beans are also a source of molybdenum and thiamin.

CALCIUM

Calcium is a vital mineral for your growing baby. It is needed for the development of strong bones and teeth, as well as the nervous system, heart and muscle function. Insufficient calcium in your diet while pregnant means the baby will draw calcium supplies from your own bones, leading to possible complications with your own health.

BUTTERNUT SQUASH AND SWEET POTATO SOUP

If you don't like preparing vegetables or wish to save time, look out for ready-prepared packs of squash and sweet potato in supermarkets. They are more expensive but if kitchen smells are making you nauseous, you won't need to stay long by the cooker to make this nutritious and delicious recipe.

Good for: Antioxidant protection
High in: Carotenes, vitamin C
Source of: Fibre

Makes 4 365 g servings
Per serving 181 kcal • 2.8 g protein
29 g carbohydrate (of which 11.4 g sugars)
6 g fat (of which 0.9 g saturates)

2 tbsp olive oil
1 large onion, finely chopped
2 x 375 g bags mixed sweet potato and butternut squash cubes, or equivalent weight of sweet potato and squash
2–3 bay leaves
750 ml vegetable or chicken stock (see pages 76–77)
Nutmeg, freshly grated

1 Heat the oil in a large saucepan and gently fry the onions until softened.
2 Add the sweet potato and squash, stir, cover and allow to sweat for 5 minutes, stirring occasionally to prevent sticking.
3 Add the bay leaves and pour in the stock.
4 Bring to the boil, cover and simmer for 10–15 minutes until the vegetables are soft.
5 Blend until smooth and serve at once with a little grated nutmeg.

• *Best served straightaway, but can be stored in an airtight container in the fridge for 24 hours or frozen for up to six months.*
• *For a tasty kick, add a little chilli oil on serving, or blend in some fresh coriander leaves.*

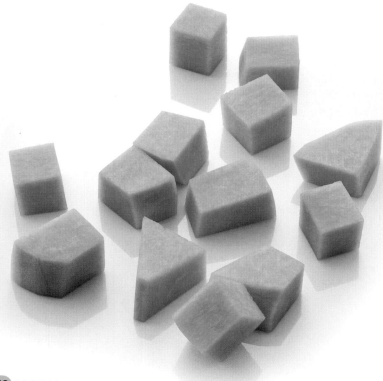

CARROT AND ORANGE SOUP

This soup makes use of ingredients that are cheap and available all year round. Make a batch and freeze it in individual portions, so you can thaw out one at a time as a quick and nutritious snack any time during pregnancy or when you are breastfeeding.

Good for: Boosting immunity
High in: Carotenes
Source of: Vitamin C

Makes 4 2930 g servings
Per serving 84 kcal • 1.5 g protein
12.3 g carbohydrate (of which 11.1 g sugars)
3.2 g fat (of which 0.3 g saturates)

1 tbsp vegetable oil
1 medium onion, finely chopped
2 sticks celery, finely chopped
5 large carrots, scrubbed, topped and tailed
1 tsp ground coriander
750 ml water
½ tsp salt
Zest of ½ orange, finely grated
100 ml freshly squeezed orange juice
Chives, to decorate

1 Heat the oil in a non-stick saucepan and gently fry the onion and celery together until just starting to brown.
2 Coarsely chop or grate the carrot.
3 Add the carrot and coriander to the pan, stir and add the water and salt.
4 Bring to the boil, cover and simmer for 15–20 minutes, until the vegetables are tender.
5 Remove from the heat, and allow to cool a little before blending.
6 Stir in the orange juice and zest and serve straightaway, with a few chives for decoration.

• *This soup can be frozen or refrigerated at the end of stage 5. To finish the soup, heat until piping hot, remove from the heat then add the orange zest and juice.*

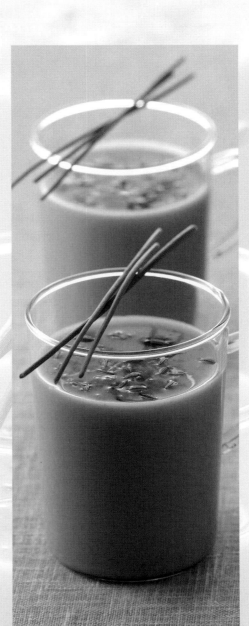

VITAMIN C

The orange in this soup makes it a great source of vitamin C, which is vital for cell repair, boosting immunity and for the absorption of iron. Stirring in the juice at the end maximises the vitamin C you receive. Combined with carotenes from the carrots, this soup is highly nutritious.

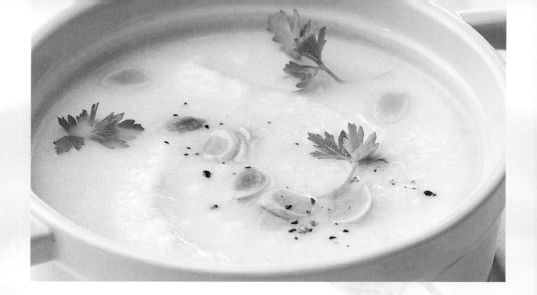

CELERIAC AND ALMOND SOUP

This smooth soup is great for those days when you don't feel much like eating. It is lightly flavoured with rosemary and its creaminess comes from the almonds. It will freeze, too, so make plenty so you have some stored for when you are breastfeeding.

Good for: Boosting appetite
High in: Vitamin E
Source of: Fibre, magnesium

Makes 3 344 g servings
Per serving 178 kcal • 6.5 g protein
7 g carbohydrate (of which 4.9 g sugars)
13.7 g fat (of which 1.3 g saturates)

1 tbsp olive oil
1 onion, finely chopped
1 small or ½ large celeriac (375 g prepared
    weight), peeled and cut into cubes
2–3 sprigs rosemary
750 ml vegetable or chicken stock (see pages
    74–75)
50 g ground almonds

1 Heat the oil in a non-stick saucepan and
    gently fry the onion for 4–5 minutes
    without browning.
2 Stir in the celeriac and rosemary, cover and
    allow to sweat over a low heat for 10
    minutes.
3 Add the stock and bring to the boil.
4 Cover and simmer until the celeriac is
    tender, around 10–15 minutes.
5 Blend with the ground almonds until
    smooth.
6 Serve straightaway.

• *This soup can be stored in the fridge for
    48 hours or frozen in an airtight
    container for up to six months.*

STORING AND USING CELERIAC

Celeriac, or celery root, is best in the winter
months when it has a distinct celery taste, and
can be kept in the crisper drawer of the fridge for a
week or so. Its mild flavour pairs well with almonds,
though if you want a stronger flavour add a few strips of
crispy bacon fried in a little garlic oil.

LENTIL AND VEGETABLE SOUP

Lentils are a great source of fibre and provide a useful source of iron, too. The tomato purée added at the end of cooking provides vitamin C, which will help your body absorb the iron from the lentils.

Good for: Preventing constipation
High in: Fibre, carotenes
Source of: Iron, magnesium

Makes 4 300 g servings
Per serving 186 kcal • 10.5 g protein
30.6 g carbohydrate (of which 5.2 g sugars)
3.6 g fat (of which 0.5 g saturates)

1 tbsp vegetable oil
1 small onion, finely chopped
3 sticks celery, finely chopped
2 small carrots, peeled and diced
1 medium potato, peeled and diced
150 g split red lentils
1 litre water
3 bay leaves
1 tsp reduced-salt vegetable bouillon powder
2 tbsp tomato purée
Black pepper

1 In a non-stick saucepan, fry the onion and celery gently for 4–5 minutes without browning them.

2 Stir in the carrot, potato and lentils, and pour over the water.

3 Add the bay leaves.

4 Add the vegetable bouillon or half a teaspoon of salt.

5 Bring the mixture to the boil, stir and reduce the heat.

6 You may need to skim the soup once, then cover, and simmer, stirring occasionally.

7 Continue to cook for around 30 minutes until the vegetables and lentils are soft, adding more water if needed.

8 Remove the bay leaves and stir in the purée.

9 Season with black pepper and serve straightaway.

• *This soup can be refrigerated for 48 hours in an airtight container or may be frozen for up to six months.*

CRISPY CROÛTONS

Make a few oven-dried croûtons to go with this soup by cutting a little day-old French bread or ciabatta into cubes and lightly spraying with oil. Crisp in a hot oven for 5 minutes or so.

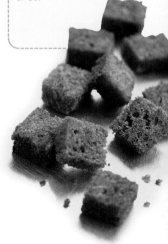

CHILLED AVOCADO AND CUCUMBER SOUP

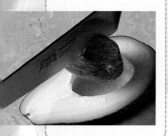

HOW TO STONE AN AVOCADO

Halve the avocado lengthwise, all around the stone. Twist the halves in opposite directions to open the fruit. Carefully hit the stone with the blade of a knife and twist to dislodge the stone.

This creamy cool soup will slip down on the hottest of days and nourish you and your baby. The yogurt provides protein, vitamin E and riboflavin which is essential for the release of energy. Make sure to choose a ripe avocado and mix it with lemon or lime juice straightaway to discourage discolouration.

Good for: Moisturising skin, boosting energy
High in: Vitamin E
Source of: Vitamin C, calcium

Makes 3 346 g servings
Per serving 237 kcal • 7.5 g protein
8.6 g carbohydrate (of which 6.9 g sugars)
19.1 g fat (of which 3.5 g saturates)

1 large ripe avocado
Juice of 1 lemon (30 ml)
150 g fat-free natural yogurt
7 cm cucumber (100 g), cut into chunks
1 tsp chopped mint leaves
225 ml cold chicken stock
Few drops Tabasco sauce (optional)
Cucumber cubes

1 Peel the avocado and place in a blender along with the lemon juice, yogurt and cucumber. Blend until smooth.
2 Add the mint leaves and stock and Tabasco, if using.
3 Blend to mix and serve immediately, topped with a few cubes of cucumber.

• This soup is best served straightaway, though it may be stored in the fridge in an airtight container for a few hours. If you want to store, add another tablespoon of lemon juice to help prevent browning, and stir well before serving.

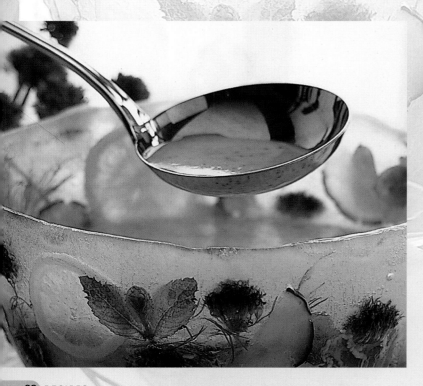

62 RECIPES

GAZPACHO

This cold summer classic from Spain has as many recipes as cooks! This version includes bread, which provides some texture, and uses ripe tomatoes. Don't be tempted to compromise and use canned tomatoes or passata, as the taste is markedly different, so keep this recipe for when you have plenty of tomatoes which you've ripened on the windowsill.

Good for: Antioxidant protection
High in: Vitamins C and E, folate
Source of: Niacin (vitamin B3)

Makes 2 372 g servings
Per serving 185 kcal • 3.7 g protein
15.3 g carbohydrate (of which 10.7 g sugars)
12.1 g fat (of which 1.9 g saturates)

1 small slice white bread, crusts removed, soaked
  in water
500 g ripe tomatoes, washed and halved
7 cm cucumber (100 g), cut into chunks
½ small red pepper cut into chunks
1 clove garlic
1 tbsp red wine vinegar
2 tbsp olive oil
1 tbsp tomato purée
Black pepper
Few pieces pepper and cucumber,
  finely sliced
Ice cubes

1 Squeeze the water from the bread and place in a food processor.
2 Add all the remaining ingredients and process until smooth.
3 Serve straightaway with the vegetable garnishes and ice cubes, if desired.

• *To retain vitamin content, serve straightaway.*

FOLATE

Folates are the form of folic acid found in plant foods. Folates are easily destroyed by heating, so uncooked recipes such as this one, which preserve all nutrients, are ideal. Good sources include leafy green vegetables such as spinach and broccoli, dried beans and peas, fortified cereals, and fruits such as tomatoes and oranges. If you are cooking a vegetable, ideally steam it for the minimum amount of time needed to make it palatable to retain maximum vitamin content.

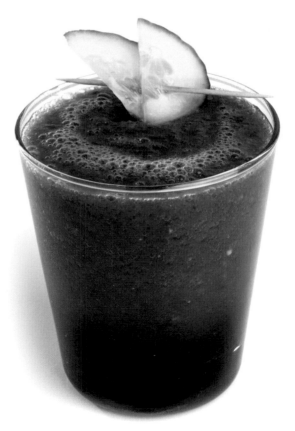

CREAMY CAULIFLOWER SOUP

Cauliflower is a good source of both folate and vitamin C. Combined with onion and potato and cooked in milk, it makes a delicious soup, whose mild taste you'll appreciate on days when you are not feeling much like eating.

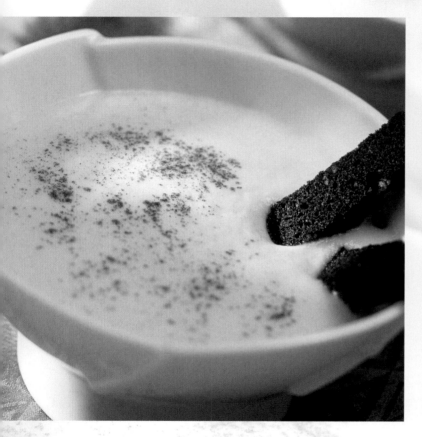

500 g cauliflower florets, or 1 small cauliflower,
 broken into florets
25 ml sunflower or olive oil
1 medium onion, finely chopped
1 large potato, peeled and finely diced
400 ml vegetable stock (see page 75)
400 ml semi-skimmed milk
Black pepper
Nutmeg, freshly grated

1 Wash the cauliflower florets and chop roughly.
2 Heat the oil in a non-stick saucepan and gently fry the onion and potato for 5 minutes, stirring frequently to prevent them from sticking.
3 Add the cauliflower, stock and milk and bring to the boil.
4 Stir well, cover and allow to simmer for 20 minutes or until the vegetables are just tender.
5 Remove from the heat and process until smooth.
6 Season with pepper and grated nutmeg to taste and serve.

Good for: Boosting folate, bone development
High in: Vitamin C
Source of: Folate, fibre, calcium

Makes 4 335 g servings
Per serving 170 kcal • 9.1 g protein
17.3 g carbohydrate (of which 10.2 g sugars)
7.2 g fat (of which 2.3 g saturates)

- *To retain vitamin C and folate content, serve straightaway. However, this soup may be stored in an airtight container for 24 hours in the fridge, or frozen for up to six months. When defrosted, if the soup has separated process again before reheating.*
- *This recipe works equally well if you use broccoli instead of cauliflower.*

HOT RED PEPPER AND PEANUT SOUP

Red peppers are a fantastic source of the plant forms of vitamin A – carotenes. They are also amazingly high in vitamin C, so despite cooking losses, which are estimated at 60 per cent, there is enough vitamin C left to make this a great source of this immune-boosting vitamin.

Good for: Boosting immunity
High in: Vitamins C and E, carotenes
Source of: Folate, niacin, fibre

Makes 2–3 290 g servings
Per serving 254 kcal • 9.1 g protein
15.9 g carbohydrate (of which 12.9 g sugars)
17.2 g fat (of which 3.8 g saturates)

2 large red peppers, cut in half, stalk and seeds
   removed
1 tbsp olive oil
1 medium red onion, roughly chopped
2 cloves garlic, crushed
450 ml water
2 tbsp tomato purée
75 g (about 2 rounded dessertspoons) peanut
   butter, smooth or crunchy
Few drops Tabasco sauce (optional)

1 Preheat a grill to high. Place the pepper halves on to a baking sheet and grill for 5–10 minutes until the skin starts to blacken. Remove from the grill and carefully pop into a clean plastic food bag. Close loosely and allow to cool. You can leave the recipe at this point and return later if you wish.
2 When the peppers are cool, the skins should peel off easily. Roughly chop the cooked peppers.
3 Heat the oil in a non-stick saucepan and gently fry the onion and garlic.
4 When the onions are softened, add the peppers and water and bring to the boil.

5 Reduce the heat, cover and simmer for 10 minutes or until the vegetables are just softened.
6 Remove from the heat and blend until smooth.
7 Add the tomato purée, peanut butter and Tabasco, if using.
8 If the soup needs to be reheated, do so gently, but preferably serve immediately.

• *The soup is a great source of vitamin C, and since this is destroyed with reheating, it is best to serve straightaway. However, it will keep in the fridge for 24 hours and may also be frozen at the end of stage 6.*

PEANUTS AND PREGNANCY

The current UK advice is that it is safe to eat peanuts and peanut butter while you are pregnant unless you're allergic to them or you are advised not to by your doctor. The latest research shows that there is no clear evidence that eating peanuts during pregnancy affects the risk of your baby developing a peanut allergy, as was previously thought possible.

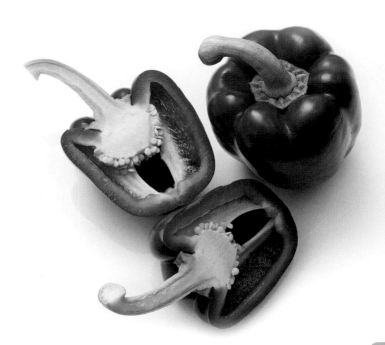

MUSHROOM AND WALNUT SOUP

This completely vegetarian soup is a wonderful source of B vitamins, fibre, magnesium and iron. Unlike other plant foods, the iron in mushrooms is not bound so your body will absorb it easily. If you want to, add a swirl of single cream and some chopped fresh tarragon leaves before serving.

STORING WALNUTS

Walnuts don't keep for long. Because of their fat content they can turn rancid if left at room temperature indefinitely. They can be kept in an airtight container for up to three months, or if you don't use them often, put them in the fridge where they will keep for up to six months.

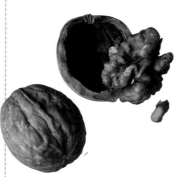

Good for: Preventing anaemia
Source of: Fibre, sodium, niacin, iron, folate, riboflavin, magnesium

Makes 2 315 g servings
238 kcal • 9.2 g protein
4.8 g carbohydrate (of which 3.4 g sugars)
19.9 g fat (of which 2 g saturates)

1 tbsp olive oil
1 small onion, finely chopped
250 g mushrooms of your choice, wiped clean
*   and sliced*
40 g walnut pieces
1 tbsp chopped fresh tarragon or 1 tsp dried
300 ml water
Black pepper
2 tsp mushroom ketchup or Worcestershire sauce

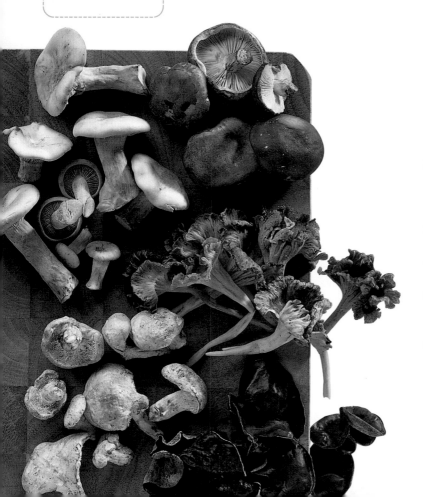

1 Heat the oil in a non-stick saucepan and gently fry the onion until just softened.
2 Stir in the mushrooms and cover. Allow to sweat for 5 minutes, stirring occasionally until the mushrooms are softened and starting to brown slightly.
3 Add the walnuts, tarragon and water and bring to the boil.
4 Stir, cover and reduce the heat and allow to simmer for 10 minutes.
5 Blend until smooth, and taste. Season with black pepper and the ketchup or Worcestershire sauce.
6 Serve straightaway.

• *To retain the vitamin B content, serve straightaway. However, this soup may be refrigerated overnight in an airtight container. It is not suitable for freezing.*

WATERCRESS SOUP

Watercress is in that family of vegetables we are encouraged to eat every day. Among the others in this cruciferous group of vegetables – members of the Brassica family – are broccoli, cabbage, bok choy (pak choi), Brussels sprouts and rocket, and their benefits to overall health are largely due to their glucosinolate content, which gives them their pungent or spicy flavour.

WATERCRESS

Bursting with beta-carotenes, vitamins and minerals, watercress is a top food for pregnancy. A source of vitamins B6, C and E, folate and iron. It enhances a healthy pregnancy.

Good for: Boosting folate
High in: Vitamins C and E

Makes 2 323 g servings
Per serving 217 kcal • 4.2 g protein
10.5 g carbohydrate (of which 7.1 g sugars)
14.7 g fat (of which 2.7 g saturates)

2 tbsp vegetable oil
1 small onion, finely chopped
1 medium potato, peeled and diced
500 ml vegetable stock (see page 75)
100 g watercress, washed and tough stalks
   removed
Nutmeg, freshly grated nutmeg
Black pepper
2 tbsp single cream

1 Heat the oil in a non-stick saucepan and gently fry the onion for a few minutes until softened.
2 Add the potatoes, stir, cover and allow to sweat over a low heat for a few minutes, stirring occasionally to prevent sticking.
3 Add the vegetable stock and bring to the boil.
4 Simmer, covered, until the vegetables are tender – around 10 minutes.
5 Stir in the watercress, bring back to the boil, then remove immediately from the heat and blend until smooth.
6 Season with black pepper and nutmeg and serve with a swirl of cream.

• *To retain vitamin content, serve straightaway. However, this soup can be kept, without the cream garnish, for 24 hours in the fridge or frozen for up to six months. It may separate when defrosted, so may need to be re-blended before reheating.*

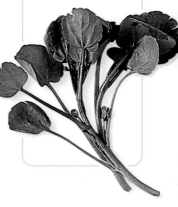

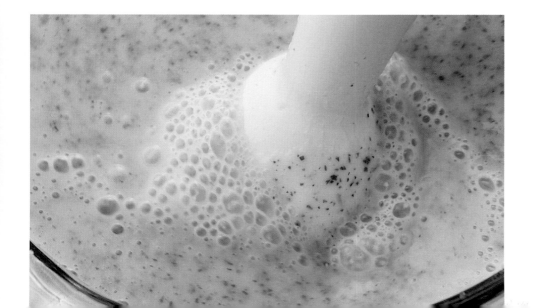

SPICY CHICKPEA SOUP

RAS EL HANOUT

Ras el hanout is a combination of spices used in North Africa, particularly Morocco, and there is no definitive recipe. That being the case you can make your own combination of ground cardamom, nutmeg, cloves, chilli, cumin, coriander and turmeric – the spices which are most frequently included.

Chickpeas are a great source of isoflavones, which are known to have many health benefits including reducing cholesterol levels, lowering blood pressure and the risk of developing cancer. While these may not be uppermost on your mind now, it is good to know that you are eating healthily for both your future and your baby's.

Good for: Lowering cholesterol
Source of: Folate, vitamins C and E

Makes 4 280 g servings
Per serving 127 kcal • 6.4 g protein
16.4 g carbohydrate (of which 6.4 g sugars)
4.1 g fat (of which 0.3 g saturates)

1 tbsp vegetable oil
1 medium onion, finely chopped
3 sticks celery, finely chopped
1 tsp Ras el hanout spice
400 g can chopped tomatoes in juice
400 g can chickpeas in water, drained
500 ml water
1 tsp reduced-salt vegetable bouillon
1 tsp sugar
Juice of 1 lemon (30 ml)
Chopped celery or parsley leaves
Chopped tomatoes and chickpeas, to decorate

1 Heat the oil in a non-stick saucepan and gently fry the onion and celery for a few minutes so they are softened but not browned.
2 Add the spice, the whole can of tomatoes and the drained chickpeas.
3 Stir in the water, add the vegetable bouillon and sugar and bring to the boil.
4 Cover and simmer for 20–25 minutes stirring occasionally, until the vegetables are tender.
5 Remove from the heat and pour one third into another pan.
6 Blend the remaining soup until it is fairly smooth and combine with the unblended soup.
7 Stir in the lemon juice and serve straightaway, topped with the chopped leaves.

• *To retain maximum vitamin C content, serve straightaway. However, this soup can be cooled and refrigerated for 24 hours or frozen for up to six months.*

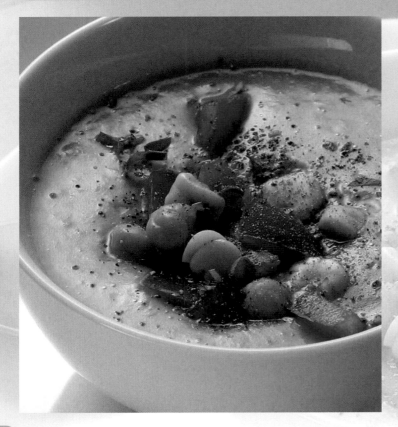

ROASTED ROOTS SOUP

This very pretty pink soup contains a variety of winter root vegetables: beetroot for its folate content; carrots for carotenes; and parsnips for their sweetness. If you don't like beetroot, simply add more carrot or parsnip or replace with butternut squash or pumpkin, which are also good sources of folate. It can also be served cold for a refreshing summer soup.

Good for: Boosting folate

High in: Folate, fibre, carotenes

Makes 4 338 g servings
Per serving 145 kcal • 2.3 g protein
16.7 g carbohydrate (of which 12.7 g sugars)
7.7 g fat (of which 1.9 g saturates)

2 tbsp olive oil
1 large or 2 small (raw) beetroot (about 200 g)
2–3 large carrots, scrubbed and cut into chunks
1 large parsnip, peeled and cut into chunks
1 medium red onion, peeled and quartered
800 ml boiling water
2 tsp balsamic vinegar
½ tsp salt
Black pepper
Nutmeg, freshly grated
4 level tbsp half-fat sour cream

1 Preheat the oven to 200°C (fan oven 180°C or gas mark 6).
2 Pour the olive oil into a clear plastic bag.
3 Peel the beetroots, remove the stalk end, cut into wedges and tip into the bag. (You may want to wear disposable gloves while you do this so that your hands don't become stained.)
4 Add the carrots, parsnip and onion and shake around in the oil to coat the vegetables.
5 Tip on to a baking sheet and place in the oven for 45–50 minutes until the vegetables are softened but not charred.
6 Process the cooked vegetables in a blender with half the water until smooth then pour into a saucepan.
7 Add the balsamic vinegar and sufficient water to make the desired consistency, and season with salt, black pepper and nutmeg. Heat through.
8 Serve with a spoon of sour cream.

• *This soup can be stored in the fridge in an airtight container for 24 hours or frozen for up to six months.*

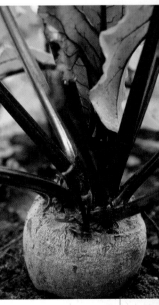

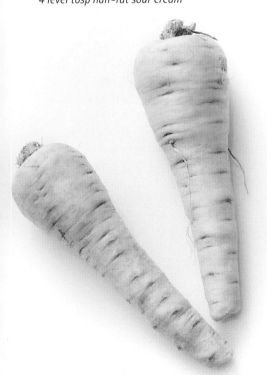

BUYING AND STORING BEETROOT

Choose small beetroot as they are sweeter and often juicier than larger ones. Also, since the leaves are edible, make sure they are green and healthy looking. Roots should be firm and wrinkle free. Beetroot is in season from May to October in the UK and can be stored in a refrigerator for up to two weeks.

PRAWN, SWEET POTATO AND COCONUT SOUP

CREAMED COCONUT

Creamed coconut is the unsweetened flesh of the coconut, sold in the form of a dried block. It is usually chopped or grated, and can be reconstituted with water to make a thin 'milk'. Creamed coconut is common in southeast Asian cooking and can cool down an otherwise hot curry. It should be stored in a cool place and refrigerated once opened and used fairly quickly.

Very easy and highly scrumptious, this soup could serve three, but the odds are that two of you will finish it easily as it is so delicious. It contains a mix of fresh spices – ginger, lemongrass and garlic, which in some cultures are said to help with nausea in pregnancy.

Good for: Blood development, tissue development
High in: Vitamins C and B12, carotenes
Source of: Iron

Makes 2–3 430 g servings
Per serving 334 kcal • 18 g protein
24.5 g carbohydrate (of which 9.6 g sugars)
18.2 g fat (of which 15 g saturates)

50 g creamed coconut
500 ml boiling water
200 g sweet potato, peeled and cut into fine dice
2 tsp fresh ginger root, grated
1 tsp lemongrass purée
3 cloves garlic, crushed
3 kaffir lime leaves
½ medium red pepper, diced finely
125 g cooked and peeled prawns, rinsed and drained
2 tbsp coriander leaves, chopped
Grated zest and juice of ½ lime

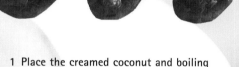

1 Place the creamed coconut and boiling water in a saucepanpan and heat gently to dissolve the coconut.
2 Add the sweet potato and spices. Bring to the boil and simmer for 5–10 minutes until the sweet potato is just tender.
3 Add the red pepper and prawns and bring back to the boil.
4 Remove from the heat and stir in the coriander, and the lime zest and juice.
5 Serve straightaway.

• *To retain the vitamin content, this soup is best served straightaway. However, it can be part made – up to the end of stage 3 – cooled and refrigerated overnight in an airtight container. It should be brought back to boiling point before continuing with the recipe.*

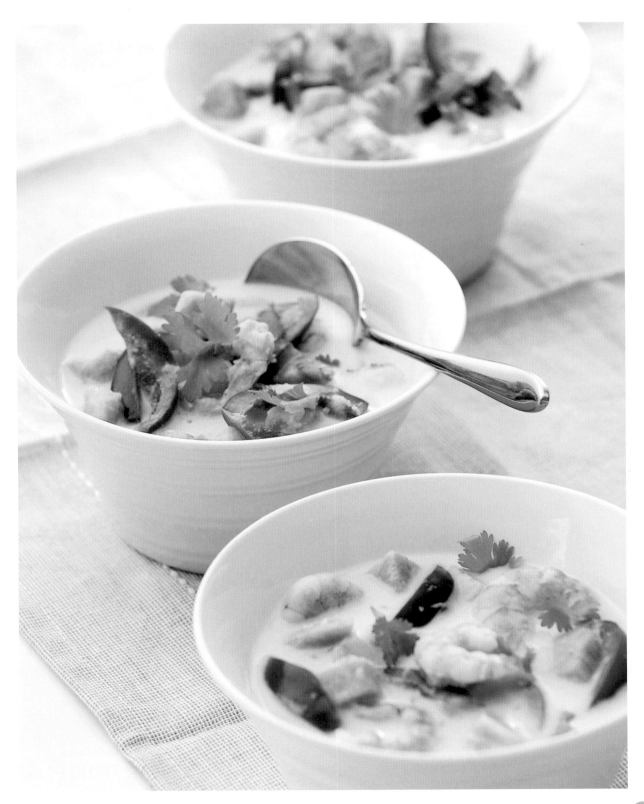

SMOKED COD AND BABY SWEETCORN CHOWDER

Containing essential calcium and protein for your baby's bones and teeth, this classic soup is a meal in itself. It is quick to prepare and easy to digest.

CAUTION

Fish bones can be a choking hazard, so check carefully that all the bones have been removed from the fish.

SMOKED FISH

Smoked fish can be salty, so wash well. Choose un-dyed fish as it tends to contain less salt and may be higher quality (dyes can be used to hide poor-quality fish). There is no need to add stock or salt to this recipe.

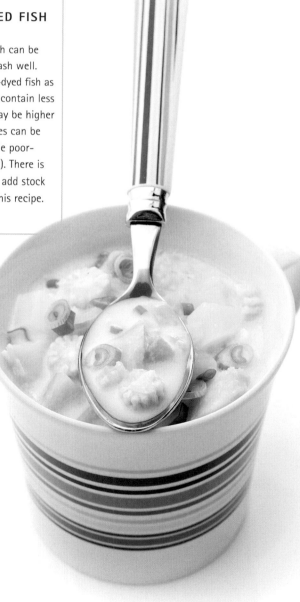

Good for: Bone development
High in: Calcium
Source of: Fibre, riboflavin

Makes 2–3 470 g servings
Per serving 352 kcal • 28.4 g protein
35.9 g carbohydrate (of which 14.4 g sugars)
10.5 g fat (of which 3 g saturates)

1 tbsp olive oil
1 small onion, finely chopped
1 medium potato, peeled and diced
100 g baby sweetcorn, sliced
400 ml semi-skimmed milk
200 ml water
Few herbs such as bay leaves, rosemary sprigs or
  parsley stalks (optional)
1 large fillet (180–200 g) un-dyed smoked cod or
  haddock, skin and bones removed
1 spring onion, sliced

1 Heat the oil in a non-stick saucepan and gently fry the onion until just softened.
2 Add the potato, sweetcorn, milk, water and herbs, if using, and bring to the boil.
3 Stir, cover and simmer for 10 minutes, stirring occasionally.
4 Meanwhile, wash the fish and check that there are no bones. Cut into chunks roughly 2 cm square.
5 When the vegetables are just tender, stir in the fish and allow to bubble gently for 5 minutes until the fish is cooked.
6 Stir well and remove the whole herbs.
7 Serve, topped with the spring onion.

• *To retain vitamin C content, serve straightaway. However this soup can be stored in the fridge for a few hours.*

ORIENTAL CHICKEN NOODLE AND MUSHROOM SOUP

As with much Asian cooking, the ingredients here are cut finely to minimise cooking time – this soup will keep you in the kitchen for a total of 20 minutes from start to finish.

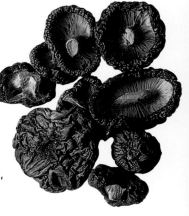

Good for: Boosting immunity
High in: Vitamin C, carotenes

Makes 4 341 g servings
Per serving 200 kcal • 21.1 g protein
20.7 g carbohydrate (of which 5.3 g sugars)
3.7 g fat (of which 0.7 g saturates)

*20 g dried Chinese mushrooms, or 80 g fresh
    mushrooms, sliced
1 litre chicken or turkey stock (see page 74)
I small leek, cleaned and finely sliced
½ red pepper, finely sliced
70 g dried soba noodles, or other fine noodles of
    your choice
120 g cooked chicken breast, shredded
2 tsp ginger root, grated
Juice of 1 lime (20 ml)
2 tbsp coriander, freshly chopped
1 tbsp ketjap manis or sweet soy sauce*

1 Place the dried mushrooms in a bowl and cover with very hot water. Allow to stand for a few minutes then drain. (Skip this step if using fresh mushrooms.)
2 Meanwhile, prepare all the other ingredients.
3 Place the turkey stock in a large saucepan and add the leek, pepper, noodles, chicken, mushrooms and ginger and bring to the boil.
4 Cover and simmer for just 5 minutes.
5 Remove the pan from the heat and stir in the lime juice, coriander and soy sauce or ketjap manis.
6 Serve straightaway.

• *To retain vitamin content, serve straightaway. However, you can store the soup in the fridge for 24 hours or in an airtight container in the freezer for up to six months.*

FINE NOODLES

Soba noodles are a Japanese-style noodle made from buckwheat flour (which may or may not be flavoured with green tea powder), or a mix of wheat and buckwheat flours. You could use other fine Japanese noodles such as udon or somen in this recipe if you prefer. Mirin, sesame seeds and spring onions are often used to flavour noodle soups.

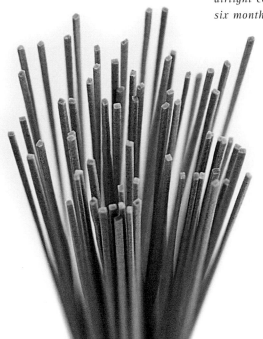

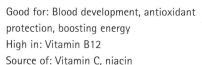

LOTUS ROOT AND PORK SOUP

This nutritious soup takes a while to cook, but is very simple to make, so once the ingredients are assembled allow to bubble away on the hob, or in a slow oven, or if you have one, speed up the process in a pressure cooker. In Thailand lotus 'root' – actually the rhizome of the lotus plant – is highly recommended in pregnancy as it is said to balance 'chi' or energy flow. Lotus root has long been used in traditional medicine and studies have shown that each part of the plant contains powerful antioxidants.

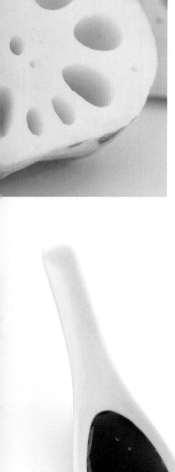

Good for: Blood development, antioxidant protection, boosting energy
High in: Vitamin B12
Source of: Vitamin C, niacin

Makes 4 400 g servings
Per serving 254 kcal • 19.2 g protein
6.9 g carbohydrate (of which 4 g sugars)
16.7 g fat (of which 6 g saturates)

1 whole lotus root (about 170–180 g)
1 litre water
1 rack pork ribs, trimmed of excess fat, and cut
  into individual ribs
3 sticks celery, sliced
4 cloves garlic, left whole
2 bay leaves
2 tsp ginger root, grated
1 tbsp ketjap manis or soy sauce
2 tbsp coriander leaves, chopped

1 If you are cooking this in the oven, preheat to 130˚C (gas mark 1).
2 Pour the water into a large pan or ovenproof dish.
3 Peel the lotus root and slice finely, placing straight into the water.
4 Add the ribs, celery, garlic, bay leaves and garlic and cover.
5 If cooking on the hob, bring to the boil, reduce the heat and simmer for 1½–2 hours.
6 If cooking in an oven, place in the preheated oven and cook for 2–2½ hours.
7 If using a pressure cooker, cook on high for 25 minutes.
8 Once cooked, remove the soup from the heat and stir in the ketjap manis or soy sauce and coriander. Serve straightaway in warmed bowls.

Note: The pork is served on the bone, but if you prefer you can strip the meat from the bones, shred and place in the bowls, then pour the soup over and serve.

• *To retain vitamin content, serve straightaway, but you can store the soup in the fridge in an airtight container for 48 hours.*

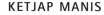

KETJAP MANIS

The Indonesian ketjap manis is a soy sauce flavoured with palm sugar and is sweeter and less salty than Chinese or Japanese soy sauces. If you prefer to keep this recipe authentically Thai, use fish sauce (nam pla), which is anchovy extract.

LAMB AND POMEGRANATE SOUP

This delicious soup is a meal in itself, providing lots of nutrients. It cooks away slowly, concentrating its flavour, and makes enough for six portions, so you can freeze some for another time. You may want to complete this recipe in two stages, making the meat broth one day and allowing to cool, and finishing the next day.

Good for: Preventing anaemia, boosting folate, blood development, bone development
High in: Folate, iron, vitamin B12
Source of: Magnesium, vitamin C

Makes 6 322 g servings
Per serving 170 kcal • 14.1 g protein
20.3 g carbohydrate (of which 6 g sugars)
3.6 g fat (of which 1.4 g saturates)

1 lamb shank (about 350 g)
1 medium onion, peeled and chopped
100 g whole green or brown lentils
50 g pearl barley
1 medium beetroot
1.5 litres water
2 cloves garlic, left whole
2 bay leaves
1 chilli, left whole (optional)
1 cinnamon stick
200 g baby leaf spinach, washed
10 g mint leaves, roughly chopped
Grated zest and juice of 1 lime
1 medium pomegranate (or 150 g pomegranate
    seeds)
Salt and black pepper

1 Place the lamb shank in a large saucepan and add the onion, lentils and pearl barley.
2 Using disposable gloves (to prevent your hands from staining purple) peel the beetroot and cut into small dice.
3 Add the beetroot to the pan, along with the water, garlic, bay leaves, chilli, if using, and cinnamon stick.
4 Cover the pan and bring to the boil. Either reduce the heat and allow to simmer on the hob for 1½ hours, stirring occasionally, or place in an oven preheated to 160˚C (gas mark 3) for 1½–2 hours, until the lamb is tender and is almost coming off the bone.
5 Allow the soup to cool enough to lift out the lamb. Cut away the meat from the bone and discard the skin and bone. Cut the lean meat into small pieces.
6 Remove the chilli, cinnamon stick, bay leaves and whole garlic from the soup.
7 Return the lamb to the pan. (You can cool the mixture and freeze at this point.)
8 Bring the soup to the boil. Stir in the spinach leaves and add the mint, lime zest and lime juice. Remove the pan from the heat and stir in the pomegranate seeds.
9 Season to taste and serve straightaway.

• *To retain nutrients, serve the soup as soon after cooking as possible. Or freeze in an airtight container for up to six months at the end of stage 7.*

IRON-RICH LAMB

Lamb, like other red meats, is a good source of iron. It is important to keep up a sufficient intake of iron during pregnancy to avoid anaemia and promote healthy blood cell formation. Lamb also provides essential zinc, which is a component of more than 300 enzymes. Breastfeeding mums need additional zinc.

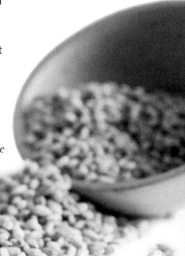

HOME-MADE STOCKS

Home-made soup tastes delicious so don't spoil it by using salty stock cubes. It's not difficult to make a simple stock which you can freeze for later use, and it is a great way to use up a chicken carcass from a Sunday roast or some leftover vegetables. Using lots of herbs (fresh, dried or frozen) will give your stock plenty of taste so you don't need to add salt, or at least you can use much less than usual – and you know exactly how much you are adding.

FREEZING STOCKS

Stocks freeze well and will keep for up to three months. Freeze in 0.5 litre batches. If your freezer is small, boil down the strained stock to half its original volume then freeze in ice-cube trays. Make these up with a similar quantity of boiling water to use. Defrost stock before use so that other ingredients cook in the shortest time.

CHICKEN STOCK

If you have a turkey carcass, scale up the other ingredients according to the weight of the original bird and include the giblets for added flavour. If you need to add a little salt to taste, do so after cooking.

1 medium or large chicken carcass
1 onion, peeled and quartered
1 carrot, scrubbed, trimmed and cut in half
2 sticks celery, washed and roughly chopped
2 bay leaves
10 peppercorns
Large sprig thyme or rosemary, a few parsley stalks or a bouquet garni
1.5 litres water

Makes about 1 litre
14 kcal • 1.4 g protein
0.8 g carbohydrate (of which 0.6 g sugars)
0.6 g fat (of which 0.2 g saturates)

1 Place all the ingredients in a large saucepan, making sure they are all covered with the water. Bring to the boil and skim off any froth which rises to the surface with a slotted spoon.
2 Reduce the heat, cover and allow to simmer for 1–1½ hours, skimming off any froth occasionally.
3 Allow to cool and strain.

• *The stock will keep in the fridge for two days, or you can freeze it in stock bags for up to three months.*

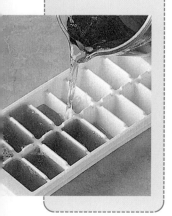

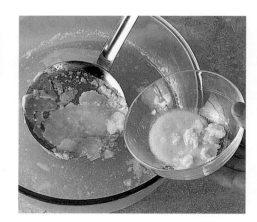

VEGETABLE STOCK

*This is an easy stock to which you can add more ingredients, or different vegetables,
as you wish. If you add soy sauce or tomato purée, use low-sodium varieties.*

2 onions, peeled and quartered
2 carrots, scrubbed, trimmed and cut in half
2 sticks celery, washed and roughly chopped
100 g mushrooms, wiped and roughly chopped
½ fennel bulb, roughly chopped
2 bay leaves
10 peppercorns
Large sprig thyme or rosemary, a few parsley
    stalks or a bouquet garni
1.5 litres water
10 ml (2 tsp) soy sauce or 1 level tsp tomato
    purée (optional)

Makes about 1 litre

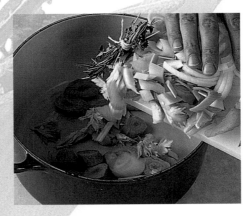

1 Place all the ingredients in a large
  saucepan, making sure they are all covered
  with the water, adding more if they are not.
2 Bring to the boil. Reduce the heat, cover
  and simmer for 30–40 minutes.
3 Allow to cool and strain.
4 Stir in the soy sauce or tomato purée if using.

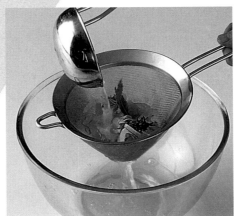

• *The stock will keep in the fridge for up
  to three days, or you can freeze it in
  stock bags for up to three months.*

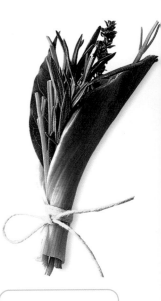

OFF-THE-SHELF STOCKS

Sainsbury's 'Signature'
stock range contains
the least salt (1 g or
less per litre). Kallo
organic ranges contain
up to 10 g of salt,
although their
vegetable 'very low
salt' contains less than
1 g. Tesco 'Finest'
chicken stock and
Marigold Swiss
vegetable bouillon
contain 9 g of salt;
Marigold reduced-salt
bouillon scores 5 g and
Tesco beef stock 6 g.

At the top of the
scale are the Knorr gel
ranges (more than 11 g
salt per litre), and Knorr
(9–9.7 g per litre) and
Oxo (8.3–12.3 g) cubes.

Adults are advised to
consume no more than
6 g salt a day.

STOCKS AND SALT

Stocks and bouillons are used to add flavour to soups and stews. They come as concentrated stock
cubes, dehydrated bouillon powders, concentrated liquid in jars or individual portions, or fresh in
ready-to-use tubs. Each has its merits for cooking, but all are usually high in salt, which is not ideal
as part of a healthy pregnancy diet. If you are used to adding salt or stocks in cooking you will miss
the flavour, so you may find it easier to cut down gradually. Either use less concentrate than the
packet instructions suggest, by adding more water, or look out for reduced-sodium (salt) stock or
bouillon, which will have lots of vegetable flavour but less salt. Ideally, make your own stocks, but
this does require a bit of forward planning so you have stock in the freezer when you need it.

JUICES

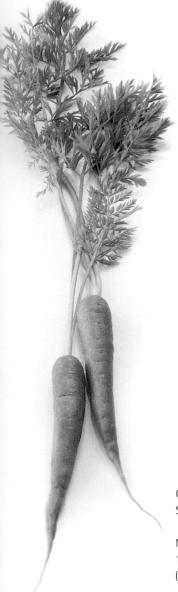

APPLE AND CARROT

Carrots are a wonderful source of beta-carotene, which helps to protect vision and is important for your developing baby's organs and eyes, too. Apples are a good source of vitamin C, which strengthens the immune system. There is no need to peel carrots, but do give them a good scrub and trim off the tops before juicing.

Good for: Boosting immunity
Source of: Vitamin C

Makes 1 200 ml serving
122 kcal • 27.5 g carbohydate
(of which 26.7 g sugars)

1 medium crisp apple (150 g)
2 medium carrots, scrubbed and trimmed

1 If your juicer feeding tube is large enough juice the whole apple. If not, then cut to fit the tube before processing.
2 Juice the carrots and combine with the apple juice.
3 Stir and serve.

• *To retain vitamin C content, serve straightaway.*

APPLE AND CHERRY

With its potent mixture of antioxidants, this drink provides you and your baby with protection at the cellular level. Apart from its health benefits, it tastes wonderful too. It's best when made with a juicy, fairly sharp apple such as a Worcester Pearmain or Granny Smith, though you may like to experiment with several types.

Good for: Boosting immunity
Source of: Vitamin C, antioxidants

Makes 1 200 ml serving
121 kcal • 29.8 g carbohydrate
(of which 29.8 g sugars)

1 large juicy apple (180 g), left whole
14–16 juicy dark cherries (110 g), stones and
* stalks removed*

1 If your juicer feeding tube is large enough juice the whole apple. If not, cut to fit the tube before juicing.
2 Add the cherries and juice.
3 Serve with ice cubes for a chilled drink.

• *To retain vitamin C content, serve straightaway.*

APPLE AND CELERY

This simple combination of fruit and vegetable is inexpensive and uses ingredients you are likely to have in the fridge. If you are feeling nauseous, you can also add a little ginger root. The outside stalks of celery tend to be the crunchiest and the greener the better as chlorophyll provides magnesium, essential for bone development.

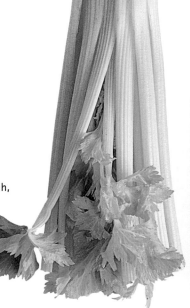

Good for: Bone development
Source of: Vitamin C, magnesium

Makes 1 200 ml serving
71 kcal • 15.9 g carbohydrate
(of which 15.9 g sugars)

1 medium crisp green apple (150 g), preferably chilled
2 large sticks celery

1 If your juicer feeding tube is large enough, juice the whole apple. If not, then cut to fit the tube before processing.
2 Juice the celery and mix together.
3 Add a few ice cubes for a chilled drink.

• *To retain vitamin C content, serve straightaway.*

APPLE, BLUEBERRY AND STRAWBERRY

This is a lovely late summer juice when the first apples are available and strawberries have not yet disappeared. The flavonol quercetin is found in apples, especially in the skin, so don't peel them before juicing to enjoy the antioxidant benefits this provides. The benefits of eating berries are endless and if you can eat them ripe and in season, you're more likely to enjoy the maximum yield of phytonutrients.

Good for: Boosting immunity
High in: Vitamin C

Makes 1 200 ml serving
129 kcal • 29.7 g carbohydrate
(of which 26.1 g sugars)

1 medium crisp juicy apple such as Discovery (150 g)
7–8 strawberries (70 g), hulled and wiped clean
80 g blueberries

1 If your juicer feeding tube is large enough juice the whole apple. If not, cut to fit the tube before processing.
2 Add the strawberries and blueberries.
3 Stir and serve.

• *To retain vitamin C content, serve straightaway.*

QUERCETIN

Apples, berries and red onions are among the richest sources of the antioxidant quercetin. Quercetin is one of the most common flavonoids in the diet and has a host of health benefits.

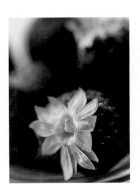

APPLE, CARROT, RED PEPPER AND CELERY

Choose a crisp red apple for this juice to complement the red and orange colour of the peppers and carrots. A green apple will taste fine but make your drink look muddy. Try a Discovery, Gala, Jonathan or Pink Lady. Red peppers and carrots are particularly high in carotenes, which help protect you and your baby against infection.

JUICING FRESH VEGETABLES

As a rough guide, a large carrot will yield about 60 ml of juice and a celery stick about 50 ml. Half a cucumber will yeld about 130 ml and half a dozen vine tomatoes about 290 ml. A large red pepper will give you about 200 ml of juice.

All these figures are guides only – yield of juice will depend on the ripeness, juiciness and temperature of the produce, as well as the variety. See also box, page 98.

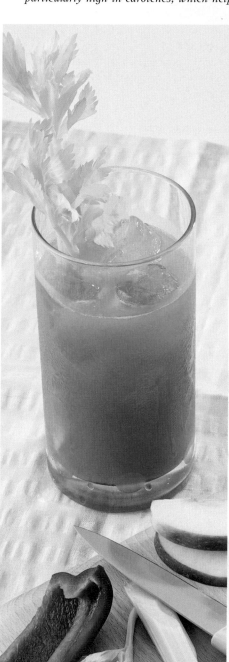

Good for: Boosting immunity
High in: Carotenes, vitamin C
Source of: Fibre

Makes 1 225 ml serving
99 kcal • 21.4 g carbohydrate
(of which 20.9 g sugars)

1 small apple, preferably red (115 g)
1 medium carrot, scrubbed and trimmed
¼ red pepper, seeds removed
2 small sticks celery

1 If your juicer feeding tube is large enough juice the whole apple. If not, then cut to fit the tube before processing.
2 Add the remaining ingredients and juice.
3 Serve straightaway in a glass, with ice cubes for a chilled drink.

• *To retain vitamin C content, serve straightaway.*

ORANGE, PLUM AND BLACK GRAPE

If you were a red wine drinker before becoming pregnant, and enjoyed the health benefits moderate drinking confers, this juice is a good one as black or purple grape juice seems to have a similar effect. Grapes contain flavonoids, phenolic acids and resveratrol, and the darker the colour the higher the concentration of these compounds.

Good for: Boosting folate
High in: Vitamin C
Source of: Folate

Makes 1 225 ml serving
147 kcal • 33.6 g carbohydrate
(of which 33.6 g sugars)

2 small, thin-skinned or juicing oranges
    (200–220 g, unpeeled weight)
1 large black or purple plum (85 g), halved to
    remove stone
20–22 black seedless grapes (110 g)

1 Squeeze the oranges in a citrus press or, if
  you prefer, peel and juice.
2 Place the plums and grapes in a juicer and
  process.
3 Mix the juices together and serve.

• *To retain vitamin C content, serve
  straightaway.*

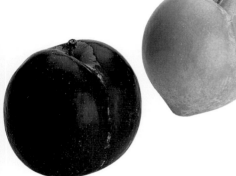

RESVERATROL

Naturally occurring in the skins of red grapes, cranberries and other red fruits, resveratrol is a powerful antioxidant. It is reputed to slow the ageing pocess, have anti-cancer and anti-inflammatory properties, and to benefit heart health. The resveratrol in red grape skins, converted into red wine, is believed to be one of several health factors conferred by the 'Mediterranean diet'.

ORANGE, GRAPE AND GINGER

A lovely juice for early pregnancy to help you with nausea, this can be enjoyed first thing in the morning. The orange supplies essential vitamin C, too.

Good for: Combating nausea
High in: Vitamin C

Makes 1 210 ml serving
144 kcal • 32.5 g carbohydrate
(of which 31.8 g sugars)

2 small, thin-skinned or juicing oranges
    (200–220 g, unpeeled weight)
20–22 grapes of any colour (110 g)
1 cm root ginger, peeled or scrubbed

1 Squeeze the oranges in the press or, if you
  prefer, juice them once you've peeled the
  skin.
2 Juice the grapes and mix with the orange
  juice.
3 Juice the ginger into a separate container
  so you can add as much or little as you like,
  starting off with half a teaspoon.

• *To retain vitamin C content, serve
  straightaway.*

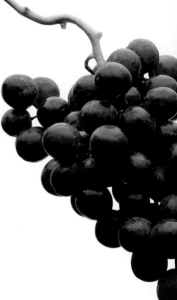

CLEMENTINE, PINEAPPLE AND CRANBERRY

You may want to try cranberry juice as it comes out of the juicer, but it is mouth-puckeringly sour, so here it's mixed with seasonal friends: clementines and pineapple. There is considerable evidence that the proanthocyanidins in cranberries provide a barrier to bacteria that can cause urinary tract infection.

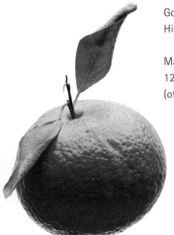

Good for: Urinary tract health
High in: Vitamin C

Makes 1 200 ml serving
125 kcal • 28.6 g carbohydrate
(of which 28.6 g sugars)

2 small clementines (150 g)
2 cm slice pineapple (160 g), skin removed
1 large handful fresh cranberries (50 g)

1 Squeeze the clementines in a citrus press.
2 Place the pineapple and cranberries in the juicer and process.
3 Mix together and serve.

• *To retain vitamin C content, serve straightaway.*

CLEMENTINE AND CHERRY

Of all the juices in this book, this is highest in vitamin C, which is found in both the clementines and the cherries. Although it may seem a bit extravagant to juice cherries, you won't regret it, as the result is fabulous. So look out for special offers on imported cherries around Christmas when clementines are abundant.

CHERRIES AND BLENDERS

You can probably get away with not removing the stones from the cherries, if you can bear the noise, but it may not improve the life of your machine.

For best results, use a cherry stoner (see page 42).

Good for: Boosting folate, boosting immunity
High in: Vitamin C
Source of: Folate

Makes 1 195 ml serving
125 kcal
27.7 g carbohydrate
(of which 27.7 g sugars)

4 small clementines (280 g), peeled
12–15 dark cherries (100 g), stalks removed

1 Place the clementines in the juicer and process.
2 Add the cherries and juice.

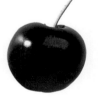

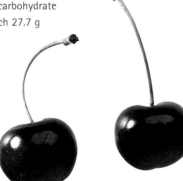

• *To retain vitamin C content, serve straightaway.*
• *For a sweeter taste, squeeze the juice from the clementines.*

NECTARINE, APPLE AND PINEAPPLE

Nectarines and peaches make a delicious syrupy juice or nectar and when in season are worth enjoying as a fresh juice on their own. Here they are mixed with apple and pineapple for more of a bite.

Good for: Boosting immunity, aiding digestion
High in: Vitamin C

Makes 1 200 ml serving
182 kcal • 40 g carbohydrate
(of which 40 g sugars)

2 medium nectarines or peaches, halved to remove the stone (285 g)
½ medium crisp apple (75 g)
1 cm slice pineapple (80 g), skin removed

1 Place all the ingredients in the juicer and process.
2 Stir and serve with ice cubes for a chilled drink.

• *To retain vitamin C content, serve straightaway.*

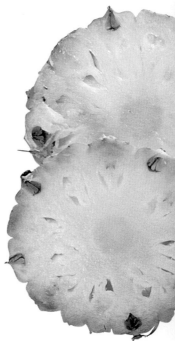

PEAR, GRAPE AND CLEMENTINE

When fully ripe, pears make a thick, almost syrupy juice. Choose a variety you know to be full of juice, such as Conference or Comice, or if you can find them, Asian or 'green' pears. Process them last into the other juice to help prevent browning or add a couple of teaspoons of lemon juice to the mix. A good source of fibre and antioxidants, the pears in this recipe help digestive health.

Good for: Aiding digestion
Source of: Vitamin C, fibre

Makes 1 200 ml serving
124 kcal • 29.1 g carbohydrate
(of which 29.1 g sugars)

1 small clementine (70 g), peeled
18–20 red or black grapes (90 g), stalks removed
1 medium juicy, ripe pear, stalk removed (150–160 g)
2 tsp lemon juice (optional)

1 Juice the clementines and grapes together and stir.
2 Juice the pear and quickly add to the clementine and grape mix, stirring to slow browning, and adding a teaspoon or so of lemon juice if you like.

• *To retain vitamin C content, serve straightaway.*

PEARS

Pears come in all sorts of varieties and the main season in the UK is autumn. Pears do not fully ripen on the tree, so are often hard when you buy them. To speed up their ripening, put pears in a brown paper bag along with a ripe banana; bananas release a high level of ethylene gas, which aids the ripening process.

PEAR, PINEAPPLE AND GRAPE

This juice makes a lovely breakfast drink for early pregnancy as it is mild and goes down well if you are feeling a bit nauseous.

Good for: Combating nausea
Source of: Vitamin C, fibre

Makes 1 200 ml serving
122 kcal • 28.8 g carbohydrate
(of whch 28.8 g sugars)

1 cm slice pineapple (80 g), skin removed
10–12 grapes (60 g)
1 small juicy pear (100 g)
1 tsp lemon juice, optional

1 Juice the pineapple and grapes.
2 Juice the pear and quickly add to the other fruit, stirring to slow browning, and adding a teaspoon or so of lemon juice if you like.

• *To retain vitamin C content, serve straightaway.*

PEAR, TOMATO AND GRAPEFRUIT

This unlikely combination of fruit is a source of folate, high in vitamin C and has a sweet yet tangy taste too. Choose ripe vine tomatoes, and if they are a little pale, sit them on the windowsill for a day or so to darken and increase their in antioxidant content.

Good for: Boosting folate
High in: Vitamin C
Source of: Folate, vitamin C

Makes 1 200 ml serving
85 kcal • 18.1 g carbohydrate
(of which 19.1 g sugars)

½ small grapefruit (130 g)
2 small, ripe tomatoes (125 g)
½ large or 1 small pear (90–100 g)

1 Squeeze the grapefruit in a citrus press or if you want a stronger flavour and more antioxidants, peel and pop in the juicer.
2 Juice the tomatoes and pear together and mix with the grapefruit.
3 Serve with ice cubes for a chilled drink.

• *To retain vitamin content, serve straightaway.*

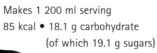

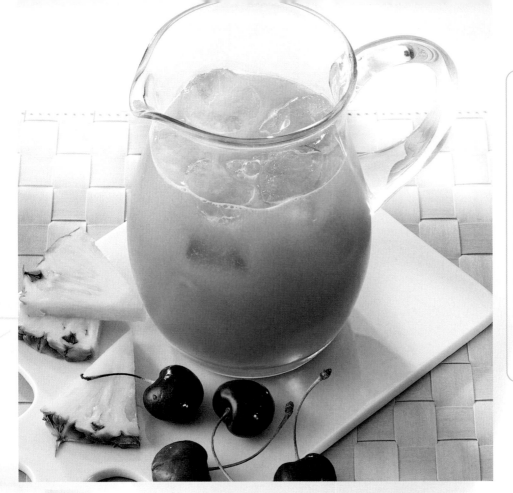

GOOD FOR YOU

Red and purple berries contain potent antioxidants called anthocyanins, which are responsible for their colour. Known to help protect cells from damage, anthocyanins help to reduce the risk of developing cancers and heart disease, so keeping you healthy.

PINEAPPLE AND CHERRY

The potent compounds found in cherries are thought to help suppress the production of uric acid – which can lead to gout, but more importantly during pregnancy is related to high blood pressure and pre-eclampsia. Keep yourself healthy with this delicious juice.

Good for: Regulating blood pressure
High in: Vitamin C

Makes 1 200 ml serving
131 kcal • 30.4 g carbohydrate
(of which 30.4 g sugars)

3 cm slice pineapple (240 g), skin removed
14–16 dark cherries (110 g), stalks and stones removed

1 Place the fruit in the juicer and process.
2 Stir and serve straightaway, adding ice if you like a chilled drink.

• *To retain vitamin content, serve straightaway.*

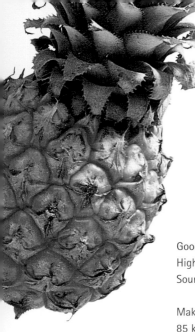

PINEAPPLE, CELERY AND WATERCRESS

Watercress is a great source of beta-carotene and vitamin C as well as providing essential calcium and magnesium to help the baby's bone development. It is pungent and mustardy, so a little goes a long way, which is why it is diluted with celery and sweet pineapple juice in this recipe. Just pack it in together with the other ingredients to make sure it juices well.

Good for: Boosting immunity
High in: Vitamin C
Source of: Carotenes

Makes 1 170 ml serving
85 kcal • 17.5 g carbohydrate
(of which 17.5 g sugars)

2 cm slice pineapple (160 g), skin removed
1 large stick celery
1 large handful watercress (40 g), washed

1 Chop the pineapple and celery roughly and place some in the juicer tube.
2 Add some watercress, then more pineapple and celery.
3 Process, stir the resulting juice well and serve.

• *To retain vitamin content, serve straightaway.*

PINEAPPLE AND GINGER

A juice with a ginger kick is great for alleviating nausea. The pineapple also contains manganese, a component of an important enzyme called superoxide dismutase, a potent antioxidant providing protection against the damaging effects of free radicals.

THE EVIDENCE FOR GINGER

A 1991 study of women with severe morning sickness, undertaken at the University of Copenhagen, found that 1 g doses of dried ginger powder were effective in reducing or eliminating their symptoms.

Good for: Combating nausea
High in: Vitamin C
Source of: Magnesium

Makes 1 210 ml serving
145 kcal • 34 g carbohydrate
(of which 33.7 g sugars)

4.5 cm slice pineapple (350 g), skin removed
1 cm ginger root, scrubbed or peeled

1 Place the pineapple in the juicer and process.
2 Remove the jug or glass and then process the ginger into another small glass.
3 Stir half to one teaspoon of ginger juice into the pineapple, and serve.

• *To retain vitamin content, serve straightaway.*

CARROT, PINEAPPLE AND GINGER

Carrots contain high levels of beta-carotene, which the body turns into vitamin A, so this juice will help you on your way to achieving your extra pregnancy requirements.

Good for: Combating nausea
High in: Vitamin C, carotenes
Source of: Thiamin, vitamin B6

Makes 1 215 ml serving
142 kcal • 32.4 g carbohydrate
(of which 31.6 g sugars)

2 small carrots, washed and trimmed
3 cm slice pineapple (240 g), skin removed
1 cm ginger root, scrubbed or peeled

1 Place the carrots and pineapple in the juicer and process.
2 Remove the collecting jug or glass, and then process the ginger into another small glass.
3 Stir half to one teaspoon of ginger juice into the pineapple, and serve.

• *To retain vitamin content, serve straightaway.*

GRAPEFRUIT, PINEAPPLE AND CLEMENTINE

Choose either red or yellow grapefruit for this is great breakfast juice. The redder the flesh of your grapefruit the sweeter it is likely to be and the more beneficial antioxidant lycopene it will contain.

Good for: Antioxidant protection
High in: Vitamin C
Source of: Folate

Makes 1 200 ml serving
135 kcal • 30.6 g carbohydrate
(of which 30.6 g sugars)

½ medium grapefruit (150 g)
1 medium clementine (85 g)
2 cm slice pineapple (160 g), skin removed

1 Squeeze the juice from the grapefruit and clementine using a citrus press. If you prefer a stronger flavour, peel both citrus fruits and process in the juicer.
2 Juice the pineapple and combine with the other juices.
3 Stir and serve.

• *To retain vitamin content, serve straightaway.*

CITRUS FRUIT

The orange is the largest, sweetest and most dense member of the orange family. Common types include navel, Valencia and blood oranges: Valencia oranges are very sweet and often used for juicing.

Clementines (and mandarins) are small, seedless and flavourful, and may be sweeter or more tart than oranges. They are easy to peel and ideal for juicing.

Satsumas are small and sweet, with a less intense flavour than an orange and easy-to-peel skin. They are seedless and can be juiced. Tangy and sweet with a distinct citrus taste, tangerines have a harder-to-peel skin than satsumas and are great for juicing.

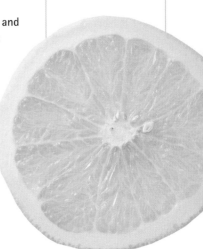

GRAPE, APPLE AND GRAPEFRUIT

CAUTION

Don't have grapefruit juice if you are taking statins to regulate cholesterol levels. Studies have shown that grapefruit can significantly increase the levels of some statins in the blood.

You can use pink or yellow grapefruit, adding more or fewer grapes according to the sweetness of the grapefruit. Juicing the peeled grapefruit will provide you with more of the bitter but useful antioxidant flavonoid naringenin found in the pith.

Good for: Aiding digestion
High in: Vitamin C

Makes 1 200 ml serving
144 kcal • 33.8 g carbohydrate
(of which 33.8 g sugars)

1 small, sweet crisp apple, such as Gala or Granny Smith (115 g)
20–22 seedless black grapes (110 g)
¼ large pink grapefruit (100 g), peeled

1 If your juicer feeding tube is large enough, juice the whole apple. If not, cut to fit the tube before processing.
2 Juice the grapes.
3 Press or juice the grapefruit and mix with the other juices.
4 Stir and serve.

• *To retain vitamin C content, serve straightaway.*

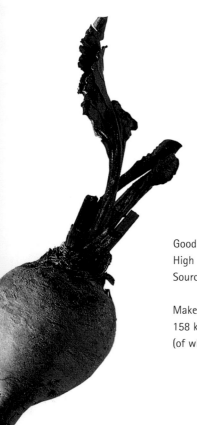

PLUM, GRAPE AND BEETROOT

This deep purple juice provides folate, vitamin C and many phytochemicals. One of these, chlorogenic acid found in plums, can help to stabilise your blood glucose levels, something that is especially important in pregnancy for helping to prevent gestational diabetes.

Good for: Boosting folate
High in: Folate
Source of: Vitamin C

Makes 1 210 ml serving
158 kcal • 36.4 g carbohydrate
(of which 36.2 g sugars)

½ medium beetroot (50–60 g), peeled
2 large purple/ black plums (160 g), halved to remove the stone
25–27 seedless black or red grapes (130 g)

1 Place the beetroot in the juicer and process first, using the higher power button if you have one.
2 Now add the plums and grapes and process.
3 Stir and serve.

• *To retain vitamin C content, serve straightaway.*

PLUM, APPLE AND PINEAPPLE

This juice uses fruits which are often available all year round. However, when plums are in season in August in the UK, choose local plums such as the sweet Victoria plum, adjusting the number to provide an equivalent weight.

Good for: Aiding digestion
High in: Vitamin C

Makes 1 200 ml serving
128 kcal • 30 g carbohydrate
(of which 30 g sugars)

1 large Granny Smith apple (180 g), washed
1 medium black or purple plum
   (65 g), halved to remove stone
1 cm slice pineapple (80 g), skin removed

1 If your juicer feeding tube is large enough juice the whole apple. If not, cut to fit the tube before processing.
2 Place the plums and pineapple in the juicer and process.
3 Stir and serve.

• *To retain vitamin C content, serve straightaway.*

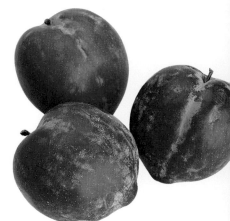

POMEGRANATE AND PINEAPPLE

The pomegranate has been regarded as nature's power fruit since Biblical times, and many recent studies have demonstrated, among other health benefits, that it lowers blood pressure. This is important in pregnancy to reduce the risk of pre-eclampsia. An all-round 'superfruit', it provides you and your baby with powerful antioxidant protection.

Good for: Boosting immunity, lowering blood pressure
High in: Vitamin C
Source of: Folate

Makes 1 200 ml serving
169 kcal • 38 g carbohydrate
(of which 38 g sugars)

2.5 cm slice pineapple (200 g), skin removed
1 large pomegranate (350 g), arils (seeds) removed (see box right) or 190 g pomegranate arils

1 Juice the pineapple and pomegranate.
2 Stir and serve.

• *To retain vitamin content, serve straightaway.*

DESEEDING A POMEGRANATE

Pomegranates are native to Iran, and there are different varieties, with some darker in their vibrant red colour than others. You can easily remove the seeds by cutting off the prickly top, holding the fruit upside down over a large bowl, and giving it a thump with a rolling pin. The seeds and juice will fall out into the bowl.

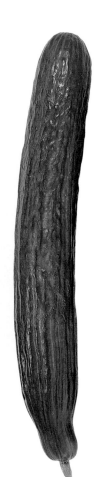

MELON, TOMATO AND CUCUMBER

Cucumber and melon have a high water content so you won't be surprised to find this a very thirst-quenching juice. Cantaloupe melon is used here, but you can use other types of melon if you prefer.

Good for: Boosting immunity, quenching thirst
High in: Carotenes, vitamin C
Source of: Folate, vitamin E

Makes 1 190 ml serving
50 kcal • 9.4 g carbohydrate
(of which 9.4 g sugars)

¼ large cantaloupe melon (135 g), skin and seeds removed
2 small ripe vine tomatoes (125 g)
3 cm cucumber (50 g)

1 Place all the ingredients in the juicer and process.
2 Serve over ice cubes for a really refreshing drink.

• *To retain vitamin C content, serve straightaway.*

MELON AND RED GRAPE JUICE

This pretty pink juice is very thirst-quenching. You may like to chill the ingredients in advance or add ice cubes when you make the drink to chill it down. Melon provides beta-carotene which is converted to vitamin A in the body. This is essential for the development of all your baby's body cells, especially the skin and eyes.

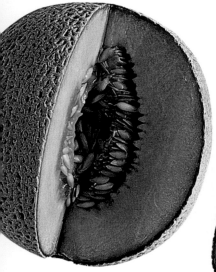

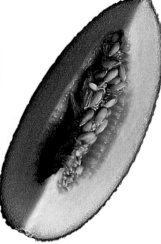

Good for: Boosting energy
High in: Carotenes, vitamin C
Source of: Vitamin B6

Makes 1 200 ml serving
101 kcal • 23.3 g carbohydrate
(of which 23.3 g sugars)

½ small cantaloupe melon (160 g), skin and seeds removed
24–26 red grapes (120 g)

1 Place the fruit in the juicer and process.
2 Pour into a glass and serve.

• *To retain vitamin content, serve straightaway.*

CARROT, MELON AND CUCUMBER

Don't be put off by the colour of this drink as adding green cucumber to orange carrot may make a sludgy colour. Cucumber contains caffeic acid which helps soothe skin irritation and, in combination with vitamin C, is said to reduce water retention.

Good for: Boosting immunity, quenching thirst
High in: Carotenes, vitamin C
Source of: Niacin, vitamin B6, folate

Makes 1 220 ml serving
83 kcal • 17.1 g carbohydrate
(of which 16.3 g sugars)

¼ medium cantaloupe melon (120 g), skin and
    seeds removed
2 medium carrots, scrubbed and trimmed
4 cm cucumber (65 g)

1 Place all the ingredients in the juicer and
   process.
2 Stir and serve straightaway, with ice cubes
   if you prefer a chilled drink.

• *To retain vitamin C content, serve
  straightaway.*

MELON AND VITAMIN C

The cantaloupe melon (*Cucumis melo*) is
significantly richer in vitamin C than the
watermelon so is preferable during pregnancy.
The French charentais melon is a cultivar of
the cantaloupe.

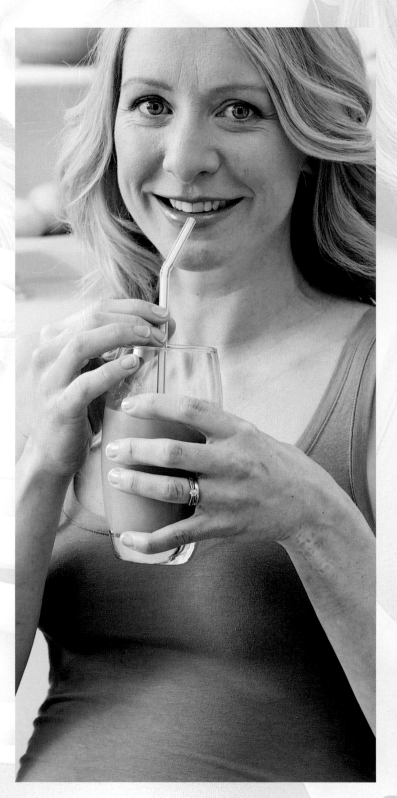

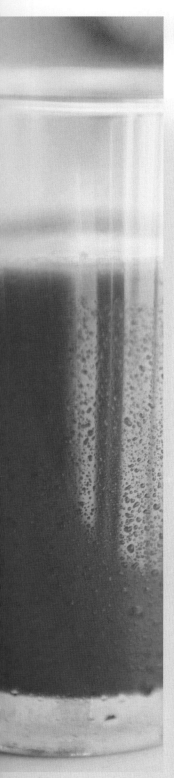

TOMATO AND ORANGE

Tomatoes are amazing in the range of different protective plant nutrients they contain, from the antioxidant lycopene to folate, vitamin E and an abundance of vitamin C. Tomatoes also contain useful amounts of vitamin K, which is essential for the formation of a baby's bones.

Good for: Boosting immunity, boosting energy
High in: Vitamin C
Source of: Folate, thiamine niacin, vitamin B6

Makes 1 210 ml serving
87 kcal • 17.4 g carbohydrate
(of which 17.4 g sugars)

2 small juicing or thin-skinned oranges (200 g)
2 medium ripe tomatoes (170 g)

1 Either squeeze the oranges in a press or peel and process in the juicer.
2 Juice the tomatoes and mix with the orange juice.
3 Stir and serve.

• *To retain vitamin content, serve straightaway.*

TOMATO AND PLUM

Plums make delicious juice, and the darker they are the richer the colour of the juice, and the more protective antioxidants it contains. It is also said that plums help the absorption of iron in the body, which is probably related to its vitamin C content. A glass of this juice also contains around 1.5 mg iron, which makes a useful contribution to your needs during pregnancy.

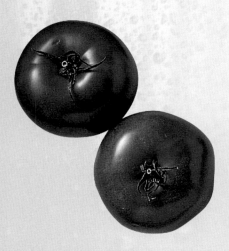

Good for: Boosting immunity
High in: Vitamin C
Source of: Folate, carotenes

Makes 1 200 ml serving
88 kcal • 18.4 g carbohydrate
(of which 18.4 g sugars)

2 large plums (160 g), halved to remove stones
2 medium ripe tomatoes (170 g)

1 Place the plums and tomatoes in the juicer and process.
2 Serve straightaway, over ice if you prefer a chilled drink.

• *To retain vitamin content, serve straightaway.*

TOMATO, BEETROOT AND CELERY

Celery has been used by medical herbalists for centuries to help regulate blood pressure thanks to its potassium content. In pregnancy, where high blood pressure can lead to pre-eclampsia, eating a healthy balanced diet is important and both celery and beetroot have a proven record in keeping blood pressure within acceptable limits.

Good for: Regulating blood pressure
High in: Folate, vitamin C
Source of: Carotenes, vitamin E, thiamin

Makes 1 200 ml serving
61 kcal • 10.8 g carbohydrate
(of which 10.5 g sugars)

½ medium beetroot (50–60 g), peeled
3–4 small ripe tomatoes (200 g)
1 medium stick celery

1 Place the beetroot in the juicer and process first, using the higher power button if you have one.
2 Add the tomatoes and celery and juice together.
3 Stir and serve straightaway, over ice cubes if you prefer a chilled drink.

• *To retain vitamin content, serve straightaway.*

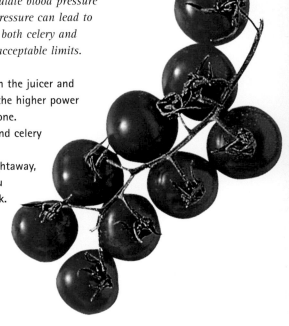

TOMATO, RED PEPPER AND CARROT

This vibrant red juice contains red pepper to make a delicious and sweet juice rich in carotenes and vitamin C. It complements carrots and ripe tomatoes and is good all year round. Though vegetable juice in the morning may not sound appetising, its benefits are worth it.

Good for: Boosting immunity
High in: Carotenes, vitamin C
Source of: Folate

Makes 1 220 ml serving
91 kcal • 17.8 g carbohydate
(of which 17.1 g sugars)

2 medium ripe tomatoes (170 g)
2 small carrots, scrubbed and trimmed
¼ medium red pepper, seeds removed

1 Place all the vegetables in the juicer and process.
2 Serve with ice cubes if you prefer a chilled juice.

• *To retain vitamin C content, serve straightaway.*

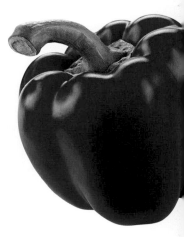

PARTY DRINKS

MOCKTAILS

Mocktails are mixed drinks that contain no alcohol. If you are having a party, these drinks will be appreciated by guests who are driving home and older children with fairly sophisticated palates, as well as those who are pregnant or limiting their alcohol intake for other reasons.

APPLE AND LIME ZINGER

Fresh apple juice and lime with a hint of grenadine make this refreshing mocktail a party winner. For a long drink double up the quantities and serve in tall glasses over ice, topping up with your choice of water.

Makes 2 140 ml servings
Per serving 32 kcal • 8 g carbohydrate
(of which 8 g sugars)

Crushed ice
100 ml unsweetened apple juice
Juice of 1 lime (20 ml)
4 tsp grenadine (20 ml)

1 Place a couple of tablespoons of crushed ice into a cocktail shaker and add all the ingredients.
2 Shake well and strain into two chilled cocktail glasses.
3 Top up with soda or carbonated water.
4 Serve straightaway.

• *Not suitable for storing.*

BLACKCURRANT AND COCONUT RIPPLE

This great-looking, great-tasting drink is a festive way to put your home-made blackcurrant cordial to good use.

Makes 2 205 ml servings
Per serving 98 kcal • 19.7 g carbohydrate
(of which 19.1 g sugars)

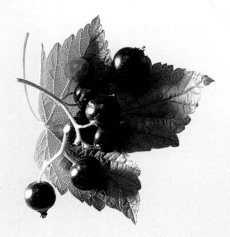

60 ml canned light coconut milk
Grated zest and juice of 1 lime (20 ml)
5–6 ice cubes
300 ml sparkling apple juice
2 tbsp blackcurrant cordial (30 ml), see page 108

1 Blend the coconut milk, lime juice and zest and the ice cubes for a few seconds.
2 Divide the mixture between two tall chilled glasses.
3 Add 150 ml apple juice to each glass.
4 Carefully spoon 1 tbsp blackcurrant cordial over the 'head' in each glass to create a rippled pattern.
5 Serve straightaway with a straw.

• *Not suitable for storing.*

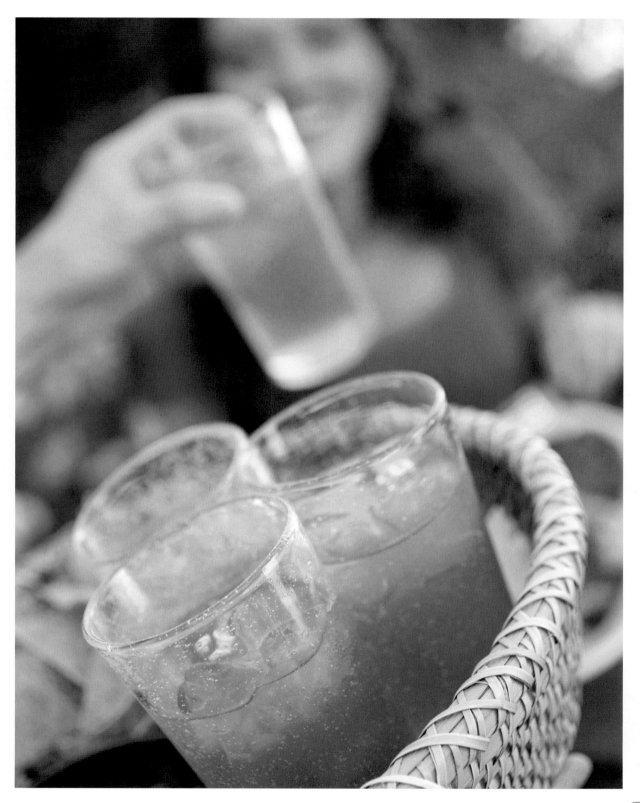

CLEMENTINI

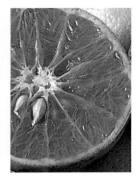

This baby-safe St Clements has a fiery kick of ginger from the cordial. You can, of course, substitute the cordial and sparkling water with low-sugar ginger ale instead.

Makes 1 125 ml serving
55 kcal • 13.1 g carbohyrate
(of which 12.9 g sugars)

1 tbsp ginger and lemongrass cordial (15 ml), see
    page 115
Juice of ½ lemon (15 ml)
100 ml unsweetened orange juice, preferably
    freshly squeezed
Ice cubes
Sparkling water
Orange or lemon slices, to decorate

1 Pour the cordial into a tall chilled glass and
  add the lemon and orange juices and ice
  cubes.
2 Stir and top up with sparkling water.
3 Decorate the edge of the glass with an
  orange or lemon slice.
4 Serve straightaway.

• *Not suitable to for storing.*

GINGER AND LIME FIZZ

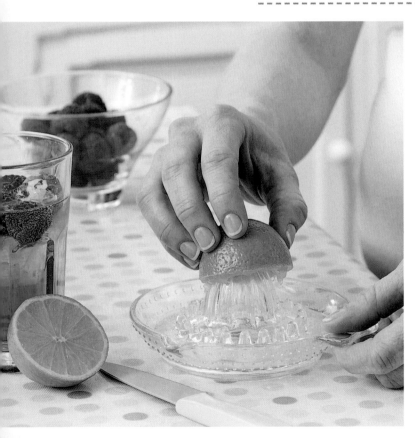

*This long party drink is a real pick-me-up.
Try it with a variety of different fruit
cordials whether home made or bought,
and if you prefer to use lemon instead of
lime, do so.*

Makes 1 280 ml serving
24 kcal • 6 gcarbohyrate
(of which 6 g sugars)

4 tsp summer fruit cordial, such as raspberry or
    blackcurrant (20 ml), see page 108
Juice of ½ lime (10 ml)
Ice cubes
250 ml ginger ale, preferably sugar free
Few raspberries, to decorate

1 Pour the cordial into a tall chilled glass and
  add the lime juice and ice cubes.
2 Top up with ginger ale and pop in one or
  two raspberries.
3 Serve straightaway.

• *Not suitable for storing.*

BLUE BABY

Using dried egg white which is pasteurised so safe in pregnancy, this frothy mocktail also includes fresh blueberries and lime.

Makes 2 90 ml servings
Per serving 71 kcal • 15.8 g carbohydrate
(of which 15.8 g sugars)

100 g fresh blueberries
25 g caster sugar
Juice of 1 lime (20 ml)
1 dried egg white, reconstituted according to
   packet instructions, see box right
Soda water

1 Blend the blueberries, sugar and juice until smooth.
2 Pour into a cocktail shaker along with a few ice cubes and the egg white.
3 Shake well and divide between two chilled cocktail glasses.
4 Top up with soda water (75–150 ml, depending on the size of your glasses).
5 Serve straightaway.

• *Not suitable for storing.*

DRIED EGG WHITE

Stable, easy to store and with a much longer shelf life than fresh eggs, dried egg whites are ideal for cooking. Unlike fresh whole eggs, dried egg white tends to foam up quickly and add body to a drink. It is very convenient to use. Dried egg whites are pasteurised so are safe to use in pregnancy, and can be found in the baking aisle of the supermarket.

PINK BABY

Pink baby is a non-alcoholic version of the gin-based pink lady, using vitamin C-rich citrus juices as well as a dash of red cordial such as grenadine.

Source of: Vitamin C

Makes 2 100 ml servings
Per serving 35 kcal • 7 g carbohydrate
(of which 7 g sugars)

Ice cubes
1 dried egg white, reconstituted according to
   packet instructions, see box right
Juice of 1 lemon (30 ml)
100 ml orange juice, preferably freshly squeezed,
   see box, page 98
4 tsp grenadine or pomegranate sherbet (20 ml),
   see page 119

1 Place 5 ice cubes in a cocktail shaker and add the egg white, lemon, orange and grenadine.
2 Shake well and pour into chilled glasses.
3 Serve straightaway, with a strawberry for decoration.

• *Not suitable for storing.*

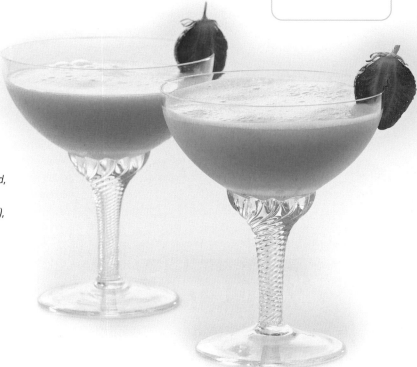

JUICING FRESH FRUITS

As a rough rule of thumb, a medium orange will yield about 60 ml of juice. A medium apple and half a grapefruit will yield 100 ml of juice. With pineapple, 3–4 average slices (1 cm each) should give you about 200 ml of juice. A lemon yields about 30 ml of juice and a lime 20 ml.

All these figures are guides only – yield of juice will depend on the ripeness, juiciness and temperature of the produce, as well as the variety. See also box, page 80.

TEQUILA BUNRISE

This mocktail is like the full-strength version but without the tequila, so you can enjoy it in the knowledge you're getting a vitamin C boost not a hangover.

High in: Vitamin C

Makes 1 180 ml serving
50 kcal • 11.5 g carbohydrate
(of which 11.5 g sugars)

150 ml orange juice, preferably freshly squeezed, see box, left
Ice cubes
2 tbsp (30 ml) grenadine

1 Pour the orange juice into a chilled highball glass filled with ice cubes.
2 Pour grenadine on top so that it will sink to the bottom.
3 Serve straightaway.

• Not suitable for storing.

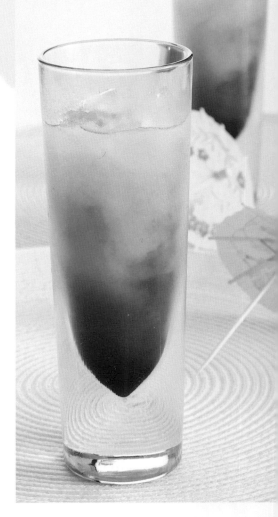

PREGNA COLADA

Pineapple juice and coconut milk are a delicious combination, even without the rum. You can add to the beauty of this mocktail by pouring in a spoon of coloured cordial, such as grenadine, or pomegranate sherbet (see page 119) after pouring into the glass.

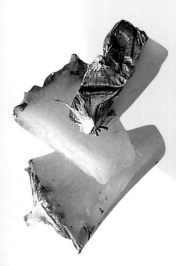

Makes 2 165 ml servings
Per serving 96 kcal • 15.6 g carbohydrate
(of which 14.7 g sugars)

100 ml canned light coconut milk
200 ml pineapple juice, preferably freshly juiced (see box, left)
Crushed ice
2 tbsp pomegranate sherbet or grenadine (30 ml)

1 Pour the coconut milk and juice into a cocktail shaker along with a couple of spoons of crushed ice.
2 Shake well and strain into two chilled cocktail glasses.
3 Add the cordial or sherbet.
4 Serve straightaway.

• Not suitable for storing.

BUN IN THE OVEN

Look out for frozen cranberries if it isn't Christmas when you decide to make this mocktail, juicing them in the same way as fresh. If you can't tolerate sparkling drinks at the moment, use plain unsweetened apple juice instead, opting for a good-quality cloudy one.

Makes 1 175 ml serving
65 kcal • 16 g carbohydrate
(of which 16 g sugars)

Ice cubes
50 ml fresh cranberry juice
300 ml sparkling (or still) apple juice
Few cranberries, to decorate

1 Place some ice cubes in a tall glass and add the cranberry juice.
2 Pour over the apple juice, and pop in one or two fresh cranberries. (If you are using frozen, just rinse in cold water.)
3 Serve straightaway.

• *Not suitable for storing.*

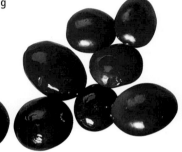

HOT GINGER AND APPLE PUNCH

Don't feel left out in the winter months when festive celebrations call for mulled wine or cider; you can join in with this warming hot punch made extra delicious by the addition of cardamom pods.

Makes 4 266 ml servings
Per serving 136 kcal • 33.8 g carbohydrate
(of which 33.6 g sugars)

1 litre cloudy apple juice
2 –3 tsp ginger root, grated
50 g runny honey
5 cardamom pods, crushed

1 Place all the ingredients in a large pan and gently heat until steaming but not boiling.
2 Allow to cool a little, which will also help the flavours infuse.
3 Serve with a ladle into warmed cups or glasses.

• *Not suitable for storing.*

HONEY

Whether a honey is runny or set depends on its levels of natural sugars fructose and glucose. All honeys contain both types of sugar but it is the ratio between them that determines the consistency of the honey: the more fructose, the runnier the honey. Runny honeys are ideal for cooking; set ones for spreading and eating.

You can heat set honey on a radiator to make it runny but it may thicken again slightly when you cook with it.

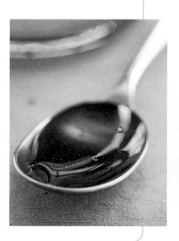

HOT DRINKS

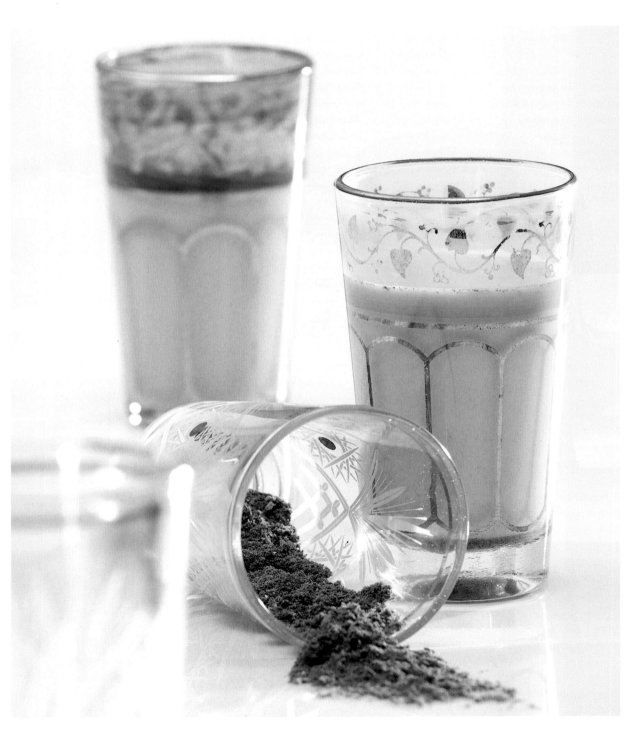

CHAI MASALA

If you like black tea you will enjoy chai masala, which is drunk the world over. It is a great drink when breastfeeding as the milk provides essential calcium and protein.

Good for: Bone development
High in: Calcium, riboflavin

Makes 1 290 ml serving
123 kcal • 7 g protein
15.2 g carbohydrate (of which 15 g sugars)
3.8 g fat (of which 2.4 g saturates)

1 tsp masala spice mix (see box, below)
100 ml water
200 ml semi-skimmed milk
1 tsp tea leaves or 1 breakfast-strength teabag
Sugar or sugar substitute

1 Place the masala mix, water and milk in a saucepan and heat gently without boiling for 10 minutes, stirring occasionally.
2 Add the tea leaves or teabag and bring to the boil. Immediately remove from the heat and allow to stand for one minute.
3 Strain into a cup or mug and sweeten to taste.

• *Not suitable for storing.*

SPICES AND IRON

Spices often contain iron. One teaspoon of this masala mix provides around 1 mg of iron.

SPICY LEMON

You don't need to be suffering from a cold to benefit from drinking hot lemon, as the additional vitamin C is great at any time. This drink uses a tea masala – a spice mix, which can be used for other drinks such as chai masala (see above).

Good for: Boosting immunity
Source of: Vitamin C

Makes 1 249 ml serving
Without honey 8 kcal • 04 g protein
0.5 g fat (of which 0.3 g saturates)

1 tsp masala spice mix (see box, right)
200 ml boiling water
Juice of 1 large lemon (30 ml)
2 tsp honey or sugar substitute

1 Place the masala mix in a heatproof jug and pour over the boiling water. Allow to stand for 5 minutes.
2 Strain into a mug or glass, stir in the lemon juice and sweeten to taste.

• *Not suitable for storing.*

FOR THE MASALA SPICE MIX

Makes about 7 teaspoons

5 bay leaves
20 cardamom pods, crushed to remove seeds
2 tsp black peppercorns
15 whole cloves
2 tsp freshly ground nutmeg
1 tsp ground cinnamon
1 tsp ground ginger

1 Place all the ingredients in a spice mill or coffee grinder and process until fine.
2 Store in an airtight container.

SPICY APPLE DRINK

This can be served as a party drink in the winter in place of mulled wine, but it's also a great alternative to your regular caffeine fix. As vitamin C is destroyed by heating, only half the apple juice is warmed in this recipe, with the remainder added before serving.

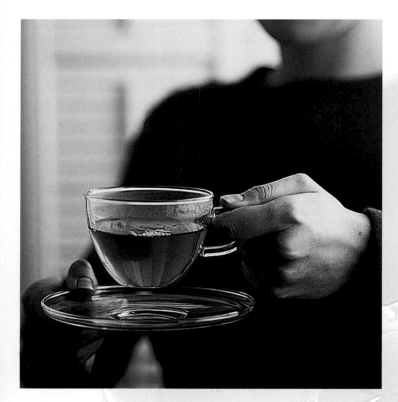

Good for: Boosting immunity
Source of: Vitamin C

Makes 1 260 ml serving
89 kcal • 0.2 g protein
21.4 g carbohydrate (of which 21.4 g sugars)
0.2 g fat (of which 0 g saturates)

200 ml unsweetened apple juice
50 ml water
2 star anise
¼ medium apple (40 g), finely sliced
Nutmeg

1 Place half the apple juice in a saucepan with the water and star anise. Heat very gently for about 10 minutes to allow the flavour of the spice to be released, but do not boil.
2 Remove from the heat and pour into a mug or heatproof glass.
3 Add the remaining apple juice, along with the apple slices.
4 Grate a little nutmeg on top and serve.

• *To retain vitamin C content, serve straightaway.*

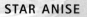

STAR ANISE

This flower-shaped, woody spice has a sweetish licorice-like taste which comes from the spice's essential oil, anethole. In traditional Chinese medicine, it is prescribed to promote a woman's reproductive health and to increase her supply of breast milk. It is also used to ensure a good night's sleep and star anise tea is reputed to help with rheumatism. Star anise is one of the spices included in Chinese five-spice powder.

SPICED MILK

A cup of hot milk often aids sleep so can be a great help in the later stages of pregnancy or when your nights are regularly interrupted by a hungry baby. Make a flask of it to have by the bedside. Ginger cordial provides a welcome addition if you don't normally like hot milk and this uses a home-made version.

Good for: Alleviating insomnia
High in: Calcium, riboflavin

Makes 1 295 ml serving
181 kcal • 8.6 g protein
26.9 g carbohydrate (of which 26.4 g sugars)
4.3 g fat (of which 2.8 g saturates)

250 ml semi-skimmed milk
3 tbsp ginger and lemongrass cordial, see page 114
Few strips lime zest

1 Place the milk, cordial and lime zest in a small saucepan and gently heat until almost simmering.
2 Remove from the heat, strain and serve.

• *May be kept warm in a vacuum flask for a few hours.*

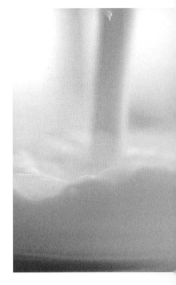

SWAHILI TEA

In the humid streets of Mombasa on the shores of the Indian Ocean, Swahili tea – a surprisingly refreshing drink scented with cardamom – is drunk in the afternoons. So if you haven't stopped drinking black tea, this milkier version provides you with more calcium and riboflavin than your regular cuppa.

Good for: Boosting energy, bone development
High in: Calcium, riboflavin

Makes 1 286 ml serving
114 kcal • 6.9 g protein
13.9 g carbohydrate (of which 13.9 g sugars)
3.5 g fat (of which 2.2 g saturates)

100 ml water
200 ml semi-skimmed milk
3 cardamom pods, crushed to release the seeds
1 tsp black tea leaves, preferably Kenyan, or
*   1 breakfast-strength teabag*
Sugar or sugar substitute

1 Place the water, milk and cardamom in a non-stick saucepan and heat very gently for 5 minutes to allow the cardamom flavours to be infused without the milk boiling.
2 Add the tea leaves and quickly bring to simmering point, then remove from the heat. Allow to stand for a minute or two before straining into a mug.
3 Sweeten to taste.

• *Not suitable for storing.*

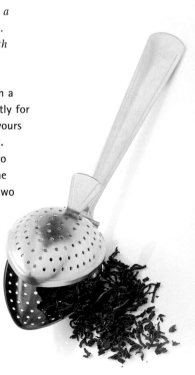

WHITE CHOCOLATE AND RASPBERRY DRINK

WHITE CHOCOLATE

Although called chocolate, 'white' chocolate does not contain any cocoa solids. Some brands do not contain any cocoa butter either (these manufacturers use vegetable fats). Milk, sugar and other flavouring ingredients such as vanilla may be combined with cocoa butter (or substitutes) to produce a rich, creamy confection with a chocolate flavour. White chocolate, therefore, does not contain any caffeine nor the beneficial theobromine.

White chocolate and raspberries are a favourite culinary duo and delicious as a hot drink, but don't use more than three whole raspberries as the mixture may curdle. Whisking it all up with a milk frother makes a pale pink foamy treat.

High in: Calcium, riboflavin

Makes 1 235 ml serving
213 kcal • 8.5 g protein
19.8 g carbohydrate (of which 19.8 g sugars)
11.1 g fat (of which 6.7 g saturates)

20 g good-quality white chocolate
200 ml semi-skimmed milk (or calcium-enriched soya alternative)
3 raspberries, to decorate

1 Place the chocolate pieces in a microwaveable jug and pour over the milk.
2 Heat on maximum for one minute, then stir.
3 Heat again for 30 seconds or until the milk is piping hot but has not boiled (the frother won't work if the milk has boiled). Alternatively place the ingredients in a small saucepan and heat gently.
4 Add the raspberries and pour into a tall broad mug (the drink should only fill the mug half way).
5 Using a milk frother (see box, opposite) or small whisk, whisk the drink until it is light and foamy then drink straightaway.

• *Not suitable for storing.*

CHILLI CHOCOLATE

A great bedtime drink, this warming chocolate contains a hint of chilli, which you can leave out if you don't fancy it or are suffering from heartburn.

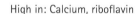
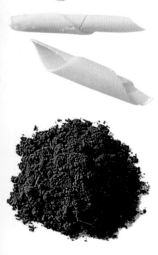

High in: Calcium, riboflavin

Makes 1 305 ml serving
Without added sugar
175 kcal • 12.6 g protein
14.4 g carbohydrate (of which 13.4 g sugars)
7.4 g fat (of which 4.6 g saturates)

300 ml semi-skimmed milk
2 rounded tsp cocoa powder (10 g)
Tip of a teaspoon of chilli paste or pinch chilli powder (optional)
1 cinnamon stick
2 tsp sugar or sugar substitute

1 Place the milk and cocoa in a small saucepan along with the chilli, if using, and whisk to combine. (If you have a milk frother, you can use this instead.)
2 Heat gently without boiling, stirring occasionally with the cinnamon stick.
3 When ready, pour into a mug or heatproof glass, and add the cinnamon stick.
4 Sweeten to taste.

• *If you want to make a larger quantity, this can be refrigerated for 24 hours. Reheat carefully, stirring before serving.*

CHOCOLATE FROTH

Use really good-quality dark chocolate with a fondant filling for this luxury drink. The darker the chocolate the higher the content of beneficial nutrients, though you will be drinking this for the taste not the tiny quantity of antioxidants. Milk supplies you with iodine which is essential for your baby's normal brain development. Using a milk frother aerates the drink and turns it into something foamy and delicious.

Good for: Brain development
High in: Calcium, riboflavin

Makes 1 220 ml serving
187 kcal • 8.2 g protein
19.1 g carbohydrate (of which 17.6 g sugars)
8.7 g fat (of which 5.4 g saturates)

20 g fondant-filled dark chocolate
200 ml semi-skimmed milk (or calcium-enriched soya alternative)
Cocoa powder and mint leaves, to decorate

1 Break up the chocolate, place in a microwaveable jug and pour over the milk. Heat on maximum for one minute, then remove and stir.

2 Heat again for 30 seconds – or until the milk is piping hot but has not boiled. Alternatively heat the chocolate and milk in a small saucepan until the chocolate melts.

3 Pour into a tall, broad mug; the drink should reach about halfway up. Use a milk frother to whisk up the drink.

4 Sprinkle with cocoa powder, garnish with mint leaves and serve.

• *Not suitable for storing.*

MILK FROTHER

Although you may be able to achieve the same foamy effect with a mini whisk, or steam attachment on your coffee machine, milk frothers do the job faster and more effectively. They can be used with both cold and hot milk but boiled milk does not froth, so it's important that milk is only heated to about 70°C.

HOME-MADE HERBAL TEAS

If you've decided to cut down on caffeine while you are pregnant or breastfeeding you will probably be looking for some good alternatives and many women turn to commercially available herb or fruit teas (see page 18). It is also possible to make teas that are less commercially available – and which may help to ease certain pregnancy complaints. The ones set out below are safe to drink in pregnancy – as long as you stick to 1–2 cups per day.

Make sure you tell your midwife or doctor that you are drinking herb teas and, if you plan to use stronger herbal teas or tinctures, seek the advice of a properly qualified medical herbalist.

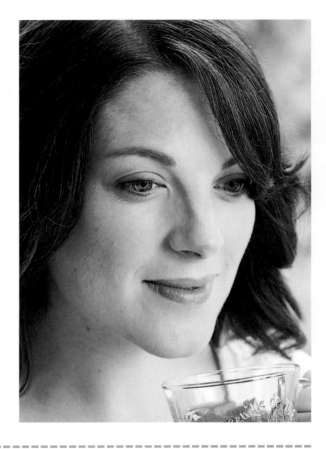

CAUTION

The herbs dong quai and black or blue cohosh should be avoided during the entire nine months of pregnancy.

GINGER

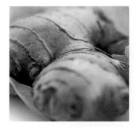

The fresh ginger root (*Zingiber officinale*) can be helpful in preventing morning sickness, though it is useful at any time of day.

Peel and grate a little fresh root (1 tsp) and make an infusion with a cup of boiling water. Ginger tea can be used throughout pregnancy, but it is especially useful in the first trimester when morning sickness is more common (see box, page 86).

PEPPERMINT OR SPEARMINT

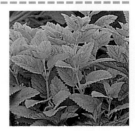

The leaves of *Mentha piperita* and *Mentha spicata* can be used to aid digestion and reduce flatulence.

Prepare your own by pouring 1 litre boiling water over a handful of carefully washed pesticide-free fresh mint leaves. Allow to stand for 5-10 minutes. Strain and drink.

Use throughout pregnancy.

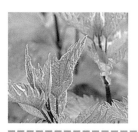

NETTLE

Nettle leaves (*Urtica dioica*) contain vitamin K and iron, which are both essential pregnancy nutrients. Drinking tea is said to improve milk flow when breastfeeding.

Pick (with gloves) fresh young leaves in the spring in a place where they are unlikely to have been sprayed with pesticides and wash well; you can also use dried nettles. Cover with boiling water and allow to stand for 5-10 minutes before straining and drinking.

Suitable throughout pregnancy and breastfeeding.

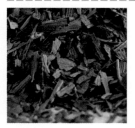

RED RASPBERRY LEAF

The leaves of the raspberry bush (*Rubus ideaus*) are said to help prepare the uterus for the birth. They also tone the pelvic muscles, may reduce labour pain and help milk production.

Raspberry leaf tea – available loose or as teabags, if you can't find fresh – is recommended by many midwives and herbalists throughout pregnancy. However, some scientists have expressed concern about its safety in the first trimester so only use after that has passed. It can be useful after giving birth to help the womb return to its normal size.

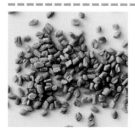

FENUGREEK

Fenugreek seeds (T*rigonella foenum-graecum*) have well-documented benefits especially in keeping blood sugar stable and helping milk supply. Fenugreek tea is widely drunk in the Arabic world to alleviate heartburn in pregnancy and increase milk production.

Steep one teaspoon of seeds in one cup of boiling water for several hours. Strain and either drink cold or reheat. For heartburn use powdered fenugreek and mix to a paste with cold water before stirring in hot water.

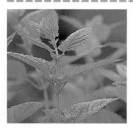

LEMON BALM

The leaves of lemon balm (*Melissa officinalis*) are said to help with nausea and bloating in pregnancy. It has long been used as a cure for insomnia, so if you are having trouble sleeping, you may find its sedative effect helps. If you are drinking it for nausea or bloating, be aware that it may make you drowsy.

Pick young fresh leaves and steep in boiling water for 5-10 minutes. Strain and drink.

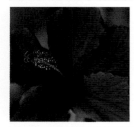

HIBISCUS

Hibiscus flowers (*Hibiscus sabdariffa*) are found in many fruit teas and are known to lower blood pressure. There are no reported ill effects of their use in pregnancy.

Dried red hibiscus flowers can be made into tea by boiling a handful in half a litre of water for 5 minutes, then allowing to stand for 30 minutes. Strain and sweeten to taste.

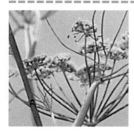

FENNEL AND ANISEED

Fennel seeds (*Foeniculum vulgare*) or aniseed (*Pimpinella anisum*) both help with trapped wind and digestion which are common pregnancy complaints. Both plants have an oxytocic effect – that is they help with the let down reflex and increase milk flow. You can chew on some seeds or prepare a tea.

Pour boiling water over a teaspoon of fresh or dried seeds and steep for 10 minutes.

CORDIALS & COLD DRINKS

BLACKCURRANT CORDIAL

Blackcurrants are an amazing source of vitamin C, and despite some being lost through the heating of this cordial, it still contains a good amount. Blackcurrants are also a good source of potent antioxidants called anthocyanins, which gjve them their deep purple colour.

WHAT IS A CORDIAL?

A cordial is a drink with a fruit base, usually sold in concentrated form and diluted with water – or another mixer of your choice, see box, page 113 – before drinking.

Good for: Boosting immunity
High in: Antioxidants, vitamin C

Makes 12 50 ml servings
Per 200 ml serving (made with 50 ml cordial)
52 kcal • 13.1 g carbohydrate
(of which 13.1 g sugars)

250 g blackcurrants
150 g white sugar
400 ml water
1 tsp citric acid (see box, page 119)

1 Place the blackcurrants in a saucepan along with the sugar, water and citric acid. It doesn't matter if you have a few leaves or stalks as the mixture will be strained.
2 Bring the mixture to the boil and boil gently, stirring frequently to 'pop' the currants, for 5 minutes.
3 Allow to cool before straining into a sterilised bottle (see box, page 111).
4 Chill before serving.
5 To serve, pour 50 ml cordial into a glass then top up with 150 ml cold still or sparkling water or other 'mixer' (see box, page 113). Stir well and serve straightaway, before the mixture has time to separate.

• *Can be stored in the fridge for up to two months.*

SUGAR AND SUGAR SUBSTITUTES

All of the cordial recipes use regular white sugar, but you can substitute granulated sweetener if you prefer, adding it to the hot liquid to dissolve in the same way. The storage time may be reduced, as sugar acts as a preservative, so store your cordials in the fridge for one to two weeks only.

   If you add extra sugar to any of the cordials to serve, bear in mind that each teaspoon of regular sugar adds about 20 calories to your drink. There are several types of sweeteners, based on different ingredients, which can be used instead. Sweeteners do not add extra calories which can contribute to excessive weight gain, and are better for your teeth, especially in pregnancy when you may be more vulnerable to lapses in dental hygiene and an increase in the number of eating occasions each day. All are subject to rigorous safety testing and are safe to use in pregnancy.

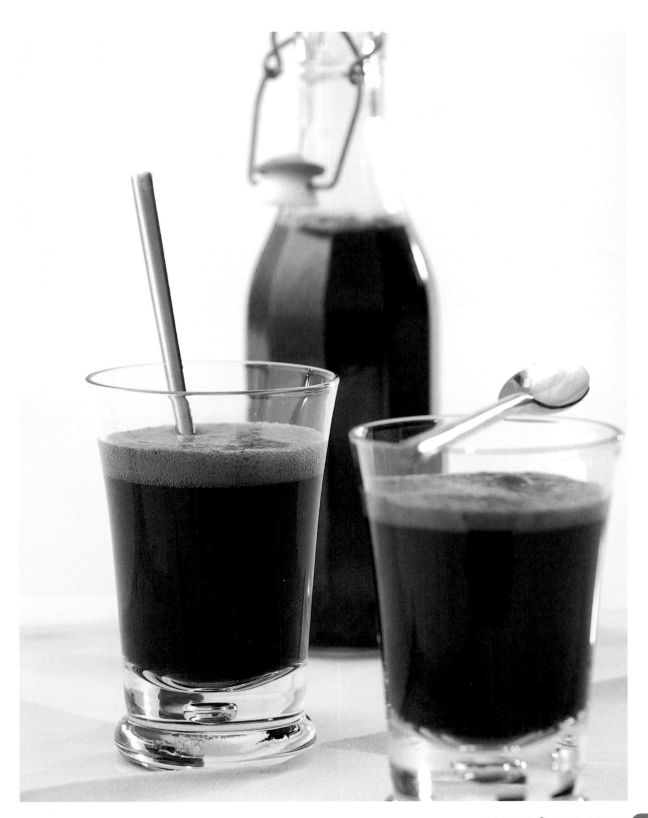

LIME CORDIAL

The vitamin C content of this juice is much reduced as it is boiled to help preserve it, but the taste of this classic is so good you'll want to keep a regular supply in the fridge.

Good for: Quenching thirst
Source of: Vitamin C

Makes 6 50 ml servings
Per 200 ml serving (made with 50 ml cordial)
85 kcal • 20.7 g carbohydrate
(of which 20.7 g sugars)

125 g white sugar
200 ml water
1 tsp citric acid (see box, page 119)
2 large limes, preferably unwaxed, washed

1 Place the sugar, water and citric acid in a small saucepan and bring to the boil, stirring occasionally.

2 Meanwhile, using a vegetable peeler, pare off strips of zest from the lime and add to the pan.

3 Squeeze the limes and once the sugar syrup has come to the boil, add the juice and boil for 2 minutes.

4 Remove the mixture from the heat, cool, then strain through a sieve into a sterilised bottle (see box, opposite). Refrigerate until needed.

5 To serve, pour 50 ml of the cordial into a glass and top up with 150 ml cold still or sparkling water or other 'mixer' (see box, page 113). Stir well to combine.

• *Can be stored in the fridge for up to two months.*

WAXED FRUITS

Fruit such as limes and lemons often have a coating of wax, which helps to seal in moisture so they last longer. The waxes used have EU approval and have been proven not to cause any adverse effects, even during pregnancy.

The most commonly used waxes are E903 Carnauba wax and E902 Candelilla wax, both of which are derived from plants and are also found in chewing gums. E901 Beeswax and E904 Shellac (both insect products) can also be used.

Generally, organic fruit is unwaxed and it is possible to find other fruit that is labelled unwaxed. To remove wax, wash fruit thoroughly in warm water and scrub well with a brush.

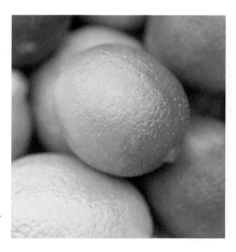

BLUEBERRY AND LIME CORDIAL

This deep purple cordial's flavour is boosted by the addition of lime zest and juice, which provide a lovely contrast to the blueberries. Research on berries suggests that the purple anthocyanins (which act as antioxidants) in blueberries are not destroyed by boiling, unlike vitamin C, and the more acidic the mixture the more anthocyanins are retained. These important plant chemicals help protect cells against damage and are an important part of the diet.

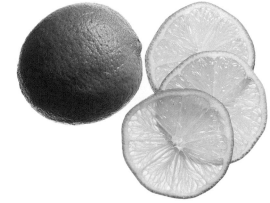

Good for: Boosting immunity
High in: Antioxidants

Makes 6 50 ml servings
Per 200 ml serving (made with 50 ml cordial)
52 kcal (109 kcal if made with apple juice) •
12.5 g carbohydrate (of which 11.2 g sugars)
(27.3 g if made with apple juice)

200 g blueberries
50 g sugar
150 ml water
Juice and zest of 1 large well-scrubbed lime

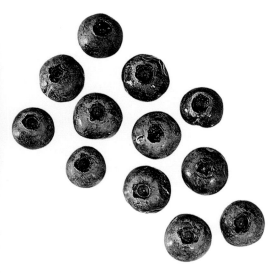

1 Place the blueberries, sugar and water in a saucepan and bring to the boil.
2 Add the lime juice and zest and simmer for 5 minutes.
3 Remove from the heat and allow to cool in the pan.
4 Strain into a sterilised container (see box, right) and chill until required.
5 To serve, place 50 ml of the cordial into a glass and top up with 150 ml cold still or sparkling water or other 'mixer' (see box, page 113). Stir well to combine. Or, for a more festive taste, mix 50 ml of cordial with 150 ml sparkling unsweetened apple juice (if you can cope with the bubbles) or still (if you can't).

• *Can be stored in the fridge for up to two months.*

STERILISING CONTAINERS

To ensure that a cordial does not go off, you must use sterilised containers or bottles.

To sterilise glass bottles in the oven place them in a cold oven and bring up to around 150°C (gas mark 2) for 15 minutes.

To sterilise containers such as recyclable plastic drinks bottles, use the sterilising tablets used for sterilising babies' bottles.

RHUBARB CORDIAL

This rhubarb cordial is a pretty pink colour and is very easy to make. Rhubarb roots and stem have been used for centuries in Chinese medicine, but its use in the West is largely limited to 'pie filler'. Ring the changes in spring by making this simple drink using the pinkest stalks you can find.

SHOP-BOUGHT CORDIALS

If you don't make your own cordial, choose an organic pressed concentrate (1 part cordial to 10 parts water is ideal). The best-quality cordials should be free from artificial colourings and flavourings.

The best-quality elderflower cordials are made from concentrate preserved after the flowers' summer harvest. These have the most taste. Traditional elderflower cordial was drunk 'neat' but this is too strong for most modern palates so it is usually diluted with still or sparkling water; some manufacturers sell their cordials ready diluted with natural spring water.

Good for: Quenching thirst

Makes 20 50 ml servings
Per 250 ml serving (made with 50 ml cordial)
71 kcal • 18.6 g carbohydrate
(of which 18.6 g sugars)

1 kg rhubarb, the pinker the better
500 ml water
400 g caster sugar
20 g citric acid (see box, page 119)

1 Wash the rhubarb and cut into 2 cm slices.
2 Place in a large saucepan and cover with the water. Bring to simmering point and allow to simmer, stirring occasionally for 30 minutes. Remove from the heat and allow to cool slightly.
3 Place a muslin in a colander or sieve and place over a large bowl or pan. Pour the rhubarb and water into the muslin and leave to drain. This may take some time, so you could plan to leave this overnight. Gently squeeze any remaining juice out. This will make approximately 750 ml juice depending on your rhubarb.
4 Measure the sugar and citric acid into a bowl or large jug and pour in the rhubarb juice, stirring until it is all dissolved.
5 Pour into a sterilised bottle or container and refrigerate.
6 To serve, pour 50 ml cordial into a tall glass and top with 200 ml still or sparkling water.

• *Can be stored in the fridge for up to four weeks.*

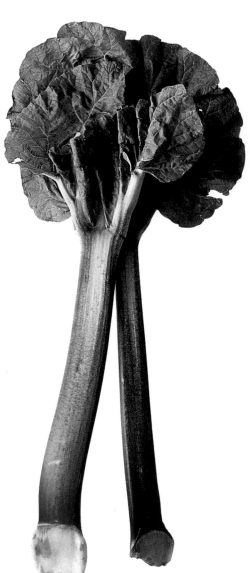

ELDERFLOWER CORDIAL

Elderflower cordial is easy to make but you need to catch elder in its short flowering season, which tends to be May and early June in the UK. Elderflower bushes are found in the countryside but their flowers look similar to inedible cow parsley, so be careful. Always collect the best, unblemished flowers only, as other parts of the plant, with the exception of the berries which result from the flowers, are not edible.

Good for: Boosting energy
High in: Anti-inflammatories

Makes 30 50 ml servings
Per 250 ml serving (made with 50 ml cordial)
80 kcal • 20.1 g carbohydrate
(of which 20.1 g sugars)

900 ml water
700 g sugar
1 unwaxed lemon
3 medium unwaxed oranges
20–25 elderflower heads, try to choose those
   that do not shed flowers when shaken
25 g citric acid (see box, page 119)

1 Place the water and sugar in a large saucepan and bring to the boil. Once the sugar has dissolved remove from the heat and pour into a large bowl to cool.
2 Halve the lemon and oranges and squeeze the juice, adding it to the syrup. Roughly chop the zest into chunks and add to the bowl.
3 Place the elderflowers in the bowl, stir well and cover. Leave the mixture to steep for 24 hours, stirring occasionally.
4 Once the mixture has sat for 24 hours, pour it through a sieve into another large bowl or pan.
5 Now line a clean sieve or colander with a clean piece of muslin or a clean tea towel, and place over another bowl or pan. Strain the cordial through the fabric then stir in the citric acid.
6 Pour the cordial into sterilised bottles (see box, page 111).

7 To serve, pour 50 ml of the cordial in a glass and top up with 200 ml cold still or sparkling water.

• *Can be stored in the fridge for up to a month, or freeze in sterilised plastic bottles for up six months.*

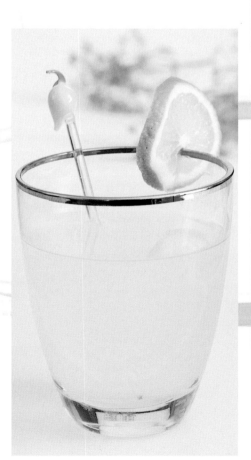

MIXERS

Dilute your cordial with still or sparkling water, soda water, ginger ale, sparkling apple juice or lemonade. The diet versions of carbonated drinks are almost calorie free and perfectly safe to use in pregnancy so choose these if you crave sweetness so you don't take unnecessary calories on board.

ELDERFLOWERS

Both the white flowers and the black berries of the elderflower are edible though neither is good raw. Traditionally, elderflowers are used to flavour fruit pies. to make jams and chutneys, and to produce cordials and wine.

GINGER AND LEMONGRASS CORDIAL

Ginger is the quintessential spice to help with nausea whether you are pregnant or not. This cordial uses fresh lemongrass too, but if you prefer you could leave it out. It is easy to make and will keep in the fridge for a couple of weeks. A tablespoon of it will also perk up a plain fruit juice. Ginger contains anti-inflammatory compounds called gingerols and it is these that are thought to account for ginger's anti-nausea effects.

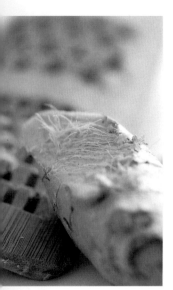

Good for: Combating nausea

Makes 6 50 ml servings
Per 200 ml serving (made with 50 ml cordial)
71 kcal • 17.5 g carbohydrate
(of which 16.9 g sugars)

75 g ginger root
1 lemongrass stalk
100 g sugar
150 ml water

1 Peel the ginger root and roughly chop into small pieces.
2 Trim the lemongrass and chop finely.
3 Place both in a saucepan and add the sugar and water.
4 Bring to the boil and allow to bubble gently for 5 minutes then cool in the pan.
5 When cool, strain the mixture through a sieve into a sterilised container (see box, page 111) and chill.
6 Store in the fridge until required.
7 To serve, pour 50 ml of the cordial into a glass. Add 150 ml cold still or sparkling water or other 'mixer' (see box, page 113) and stir well.

• *Can be stored in the fridge for up to two weeks.*

LEMONGRASS

Lemongrass is a herb with a strong citrusy flavour. A staple of southeast Asian cooking, it is becoming more available in UK supermarkets. Choose firm and heavy stalks, with no bruising. If it feels light, it may have dried out too much. For the best result, use only the lower 10–15 cm of the stalk, discarding the upper fibrous part. Bruise the stem to release the flavour before chopping. Soak dried stalks in hot water before using in the same way. If you can't find fresh lemongrass, purée is available in jars or tubes from the supermarket.

FRESH RASPBERRY AND APPLE DRINK

Raspberries contain folate, which is so important in early pregnancy, and they are simply prepared here to maximise their nutritional value. Added to pressed apple juice they make a delicious summer drink. If you have a juicer, you can make your own apple juice, but otherwise, choose a good-quality unsweetened one.

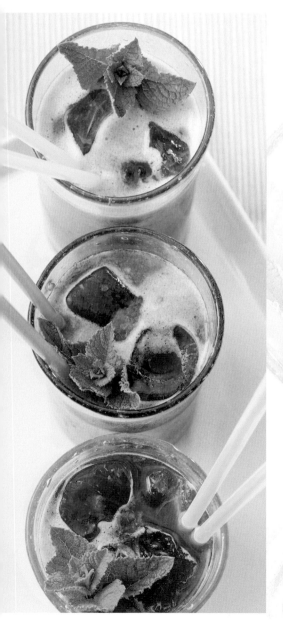

Good for: Boosting folate
High in: Vitamin C
Source of: Folate

Makes 2 225 ml servings
Per serving
58 kcal • 12.7 g carbohydrate
(of which 12.7 g sugars)

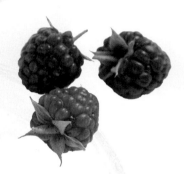

150 g raspberries
150 ml water
200 ml unsweetened apple juice
Ice cubes, to serve

1 Place the raspberries and water in a blender and process lightly.
2 Strain the raspberry mixture through a sieve over a bowl to remove the pips.
3 Mix in the apple juice and stir well to combine. Pour into glasses over ice.

• *To retain vitamin content, serve straightaway.*

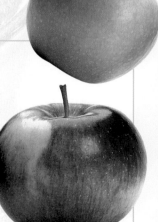

APPLES

Among the English apple cultivars to try are: 'James Grieve'; 'Discovery' which has a crisp texture, sharp taste and red skin; 'Lord Lambourne', a thin-skinned green apple; 'Cox's Orange Pippin', probably the most popular dessert apple; 'Worcester Pearmain'; and the cooking apple 'Bramley's Seedling'.

FRESH LEMONADE

This quick recipe uses the whole lemon, so you will benefit from the antioxidant limonenes and flavonoids found in the pith and zest in addition to the nutrients contained in the juice. You can drink it as it is over ice, or in French pressé style, which means stirring in more water and sugar or sugar substitute to taste.

Good for: Boosting immunity, quenching thirst
High in: Vitamin C

Makes 2 125 ml servings
Per serving 117 kcal • 27.7 g carbohydrate
(of which 27.7 g sugars)

50 g white sugar
100 ml boiling water
1 large, unwaxed lemon, washed
100 ml cold water
Ice cubes, to serve

1 Place the sugar in a bowl and pour over the boiling water. Stir until the sugar has all dissolved.
2 Cut the lemon into 8 pieces and place in a blender or processor with 100 ml water, and blitz until the lemon is finely chopped.
3 Strain the mixture through a sieve over a jug, pressing the fruit well to squeeze out all the liquid.
4 Add the sugar syrup and stir well.
5 To serve, pour half the mixture into a glass, add a handful of ice cubes and additional chilled water or soda water as required.

• *To retain vitamin C content, serve straightaway.*

ZESTS

The coloured outer layer of citrus fruit like oranges, lemons, limes and grapefruit contains essential oils packed with nutrients. Rather than lose their goodness when cooking, it is possible to remove the zest in a number of ways. A vegetable peeler or special zesting tool (usually with a stainless steel rectangular head and five holes) can remove strips or fine shavings of zest while a hollow box or microplane grater can be used when a sprinkling is required.

Zests can be bitter so if you are juicing a whole citrus fruit, you may prefer to remove the skin first (unless you want a real 'tang'), although you do then lose some of the nutrients. Alternatively juice the whole fruit zest and all and add a little sugar substitute to taste.

FRESH ORANGEADE

This recipe uses thin-skinned juicing oranges and, as with the fresh lemonade (see opposite), since the whole orange is used, you have all the benefits of the nutrients in the pith and zest as well as the juice. You can drink it as it is over ice, or pressé style, in which you add more water or sugar or sugar substitute as desired. For an extra kick, add lemon or lime juice, or a spoonful of ginger cordial.

Good for: Boosting immunity
High in: Vitamin C
Source of: Folate

Makes 2 220 ml servings
Per serving 119 kcal • 28.3 g carbohydrate
(of which 28.3 g sugars)

40 g white sugar
150 ml boiling water
2 medium, thin-skinned or juicing oranges
  (300 g), well scrubbed
150 ml water

1 Place the sugar in a bowl and pour over the boiling water. Stir until the sugar has all dissolved.
2 Cut the oranges into 8 pieces and place in the processor with 150 ml water, and blitz until the oranges are finely chopped.
3 Strain the mixture through a sieve over a jug, pressing the fruit well to squeeze out all the liquid.
4 Add the sugar syrup and stir well.

• *To retain vitamin C content, serve straightaway.*

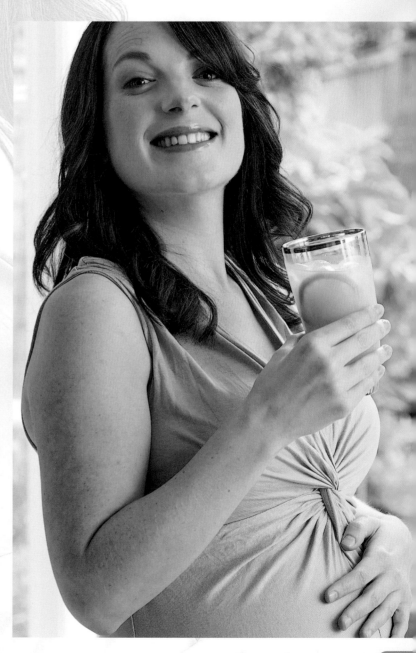

ICED TEA

A really refreshing drink during the summer months, this can be made with decaffeinated or regular teabags but remember not to drink too much caffeine. This drink makes enough for two, so keep some chilling in the fridge. The vitamin C content is useful for maintaining a strong immune system.

ICED TEA THE WORLD OVER

Popular in Europe, North America and the Far East, iced tea is a traditional summer drink made from the steeped leaves of the tea plant (*Camellia sinensis*) flavoured with fruit. In addition to the lemon and oranges used in this recipe, peach, raspberry, lime, passion fruit and cherry are popular additions. Whatever you choose, serve well chilled with plenty of ice cubes.

Good for: Boosting immunity, quenching thirst
High in: Vitamin C

Makes 2 270 ml servings
Per serving 50 kcal • 12.1 g carbohydrate
(of which 12.1 g sugars)

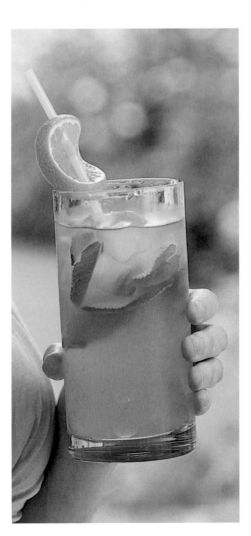

1 teabag
400 ml boiling water
4 tsp sugar
2 tbsp lemon juice
100 ml freshly squeezed orange juice (about 2 medium oranges)
Mint leaves
Ice cubes

1 Place the teabag in a measuring jug and pour over the boiling water. Allow to brew for 5 minutes before removing the bag. Stir in the sugar.
2 Chill until required.
3 To serve, for each portion, pour half the tea mixture into a glass and add 1 tbsp lemon juice and 50 ml freshly squeezed orange juice. Stir well to combine and then add some mint leaves and a handful of ice cubes.

• *To retain vitamin C content make and chill the tea in advance, but once the juices are added serve straightaway.*

POMEGRANATE SHERBERT

The word sherbet came originally from Arabia, where it meant a cool drink made from sweetened fruit juices, spices and sometimes rose petals. These drinks were often cooled with ice and over time, frozen sorbets or sherbets came to be eaten to cleanse the palate, and in Europe the word came to mean a frozen dessert. Here is a beautiful red sherbet made from fresh pomegranate juice, which is delicious poured over ice and topped up with still or sparkling water.

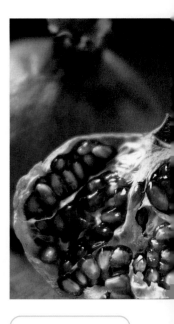

Good for: Quenching thirst, cleansing the palate
Source of: Antioxidants

Makes 8 50 ml servings
Per 200 ml serving (made with 50 ml sherbet)
59 kcal • 14.7 g carbohydrate
(of which 14.7 g sugars)

2 large red pomegranates, or around 320 g pomegranate arils (seeds)
100 g white sugar
200 ml water
½ tsp citric acid (see box, right)

1 Juice the pomegranates or press the seeds through a sieve to extract the juice.
2 Boil the sugar, citric acid and water together in a saucepan, and when the sugar has dissolved, add the pomegranate juice.
3 Boil for another 2 minutes before removing from the heat then let the mixture cool.
4 Once cool, pour into a sterilised container (see box, right) and refrigerate before use.
5 To serve, pour 50 ml of the pomegranate mixture into a glass and top with 150 ml still or sparkling water.

• *Can be stored in a sealed container in the fridge for up to two months.*

CITRIC ACID

Citric acid is used in the cordial recipes for its qualities as a preservative. It occurs naturally in the greatest quantity in lemons and limes but all citrus fruits contain significant amounts. Citric acid can be bought in pharmacies and online.

HOME-MADE ICE LOLLIES

For hot summer days, ice lollies are ideal for quenching thirst and refreshing your mouth. Use freshly squeezed or pressed juices, diluted with water and freeze in ice-lolly moulds.

USING LOLLY MOULDS
1 Squeeze or press a juice of your choice.
2 Dilute with water and sweeten to taste.
3 Pour into ice-lolly moulds and clip the tops on.
4 Freeze for several hours then eat direct from the freezer.

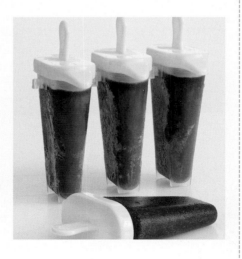

Page	Description	Single portion	Energy kcal	Protein g	Carbo-hydrate g	Sugars g	Fat g	Saturates g	Fibre g	Sodium mg	Salt g
						MAJOR NUTRIENTS					
36	**SMOOTHIES & SHAKES**	ml									
36	Mango and passion fruit smoothie	230	141	1.7	32.7	29.6	0.5	0.3	3.1	13	0.03
38	Mango, apricot and pineapple smoothie	280	163	2.4	37.1	36.8	0.5	0	7.1	15	0.04
38	Mango and peach smoothie	310	130	1.6	30	29.6	0.4	0	5.8	5	0.01
39	Tropical delight smoothie	275	104	1.4	23.4	22.4	0.5	0.2	1.8	110	0.28
40	Nectarine, raspberry and orange smoothie	360	113	3.7	23.8	23.8	0.4	0	7.7	6	0.02
41	Vanilla, banana and prune smoothie	285	318	10.1	34	32	15.7	10.3	4.1	103	0.26
41	Spicy prune and apple smoothie	355	238	7	49	47.4	1.6	0.8	5.9	73	0.18
42	Cherry heaven	275	178	7.5	16.1	16.1	9.3	5.2	3.7	74	0.19
43	Raspberry, pomegranate and papaya smoothie	295	108	1.8	24.3	24.3	0.3	0	7.3	9	0.02
44	Nectarine and passion fruit smoothie	400	204	8.5	39	37.1	1.5	0.8	7.4	71	0.18
45	Berry boost smoothie	275	98	5.8	16	15.7	1.2	0.7	3.7	71	0.18
46	Red breakfast smoothie (with pear)	260	77	1.3	17.3	17.3	0.2	0	3.7	13	0.03
46	Red breakfast smoothie (with banana)	215	91	1.6	20.4	19.6	0.3	0	3.3	12	0.03
46	Summer fruits smoothie	275	88	1.6	19.4	19.4	0.4	0	8.7	7	0.02
47	Date and almond smoothie	275	145	7.6	19.7	19.1	4	0.7	3.2	114	0.29
47	Kiwi, pear and grape smoothie	350	147	2	33.1	32.7	0.8	0	5.4	15	0.04
48	Kiwi, apple and banana smoothie	320	178	2.3	40.4	38.1	0.8	0	4.6	7	0.02
48	Grape, pineapple and and banana smoothie	310	179	1.6	42.1	40.5	0.4	0	2.9	11	0.03
49	Pineapple, banana, and ginger smoothie	320	161	1.5	37.5	35.6	0.6	0	3.2	11	0.03
50	Papaya, grape and pear smoothie	295	106	1	24.9	24.9	0.3	0	3.8	13	0.03
50	Papaya and strawberry smoothie	340	102	1.8	23.1	23.1	0.3	0.0	4.1	21	0.05
51	Strawberry milkshake	260	165	5.8	23.3	23.2	5.5	3.4	2.4	109	0.27
51	Dairy-free strawberry milkshake	280	138	1.2	30.3	24.1	1.3	0	3.5	63	0.16
52	Chocolate surprise shake	255	215	7.9	29.1	27.7	7.5	3.9	2.1	168	0.42
52	Spiced mint lassi	205	114	9.6	14.3	13.5	2	1.4	0	127	0.32
53	Mango lassi	250	128	7.6	20.5	19.9	1.7	1.1	2.8	96	0.24
54	**SOUPS**	g									
54	Pea and spinach	350	120	8.4	12.2	4.5	4.2	0.5	7.2	25	0.06
56	Creamy green pepper	333	193	8.6	18.8	14.6	9.3	3.2	4.3	171	0.43
57	Billion beans and garlic	384	268	15.6	28	4.6	10.3	3.4	9.2	538	1.35
58	Butternut squash and sweet potato	365	181	2.8	29	11.4	6	0.9	5.1	49	0.12
59	Carrot and orange	293	84	1.5	12.3	11.1	3.2	0.3	4.6	330	0.83
60	Celeriac and almond	344	178	6.5	7	4.9	13.7	1.3	4.8	280	0.7
61	Lentil and vegetable	299	186	10.5	30.6	5.2	3.6	0.5	6.7	256	0.64
62	Chilled avocado and cucumber	346	237	7.5	8.6	6.9	19.1	3.5	5.4	91	0.23
63	Gazpacho	372	185	3.7	15.3	10.7	12.1	1.9	4.7	96	0.24
64	Creamy cauliflower	335	170	9.1	17.3	10.2	7.2	2.3	4.5	126	0.32
65	Hot red pepper and peanut	290	254	9.1	15.9	12.9	17.2	3.8	5.6	118	0.3
66	Mushroom and walnut	315	238	9.2	4.8	3.4	19.9	2	3.3	69	0.17
67	Watercress	323	217	4.2	10.5	7.1	14.7	2.7	2.3	582	1.46
68	Spicy chickpea	280	127	6.4	16.4	6.4	4.1	0.3	5.3	64	0.16
69	Roasted roots	338	145	2.3	16.7	12.7	7.7	1.9	6.1	247	0.62
70	Prawn, sweet potato and coconut	430	334	18	24.5	9.6	18.2	15	4.3	1044	2.61
72	Smoked cod and baby sweetcorn chowder	470	352	28.4	35.9	14.4	10.5	3	4.1	1229	3.07
73	Oriental chicken noodle and mushroom	341	200	21.1	20.7	5.3	3.7	0.7	2.5	187	0.47
74	Lotus root and pork	400	254	19.2	6.9	4	16.7	6	3.2	227	0.57
75	Lamb and pomegranate	322	170	14.1	20.3	6	3.6	1.4	5.5	80	0.2
76	**HOME-MADE STOCKS**	ml									
76	Chicken	500	7	0.7	0.4	0.3	0.3	0.1	0	0	0
77	Vegetable	500	3	0.1	0.5	0.4	trace	trace	0	0	0
78	**JUICES**	ml									
78	Apple and carrot	200	122	1.5	27.5	26.7	0.7	0.2	9.4	45	0.11
78	Apple and cherry	200	121	1.4	28.3	28.3	0.3	0	7.5	5	0.01
79	Apple and celery	200	71	1.1	15.9	15.9	0.4	0	5.8	75	0.19
79	Apple, blueberry and strawberry	200	129	1.5	29.7	26.1	0.5	0	7.3	7	0.02
80	Apple, carrot, red pepper and celery	225	99	1.8	21.4	20.9	0.7	0.1	7.8	62	0.16

Carotene mcg	Thiamin mg	Riboflavin mg	Niacin mg	Folate mcg	Vitamin C mg	Vitamin E mg	Vitamin B6 mg	Vitamin B12 mcg	Calcium mg	Iron mg	Potassium mg	Magnesium mg	Iodine mcg	Phosphorus mg	Copper mg	Selenium mcg
2701	0.06	0.08	0.8	0	59	1.58	0.19	0	18.9	1.1	281	21	0	25.2	0.19	0
1040	0.1	0.13	1.4	10	58	1.35	0.26	0	45.9	2.1	691	35.7	0	45.9	0.28	3
948	0.08	0.11	1.1	6	80	1.3	0.2	0	25.4	1.2	431	28.2	3	39.5	0.2	0
15	0.1	0.1	0.8	10	24	0.23	0.25	0	37.5	0.5	550	52.5	5	45	0.1	0
192	0.13	0.13	1.5	52	127	0.52	0.16	0	42.3	1.4	562	42.3	7	78	0.16	3
60	0.23	0.29	1.1	21	9	0.78	0.31	0.3	202.8	1.2	824	54.6	65	252.2	0.13	5
100	0.22	0.39	1.4	32	22	0.16	0.32	0.3	199	2	1043	57.8	39	211.9	0.19	3
75	0.08	0.4	0.5	15	20	0.5	0.13	0.2	170	0.8	405	25	0	157.5	0.1	3
1009	0.09	0.12	0.9	27	104	0.35	0.38	0	50.2	1.3	566	29.5	0	47.2	0.24	0
414	0.18	0.36	2	29	72	0.22	0.29	0.3	180	1.3	864	68.4	43	216	0.22	4
23	0.18	0.28	0.9	40	87	0.2	0.1	0.3	185	0.7	433	27.5	43	175	0.15	3
19	0.07	0.05	0.9	26	104	0.63	0.09	0	32.9	0.7	324	21.2	9	40	0.12	0
17	0.09	0.06	1	30	105	0.45	0.19	0	28	0.7	396	30.1	13	43	0.11	2
48	0.05	0.1	0.7	30	87	0.6	0.1	0	47.5	1.1	425	27.5	0	50	0.18	0
10	0.03	0.25	0.4	13	7	0	0.05	0.8	252.5	0.2	205	12.5	0	15	0.05	0
67	0.03	0.06	0.7	3	77	0	0.26	0	60.8	1.6	554	32	0	64	0.22	0
58	0.06	0.09	1.1	17	78	0.26	0.44	0	34.8	0.8	771	52.2	9	63.8	0.2	0
42	0.14	0.06	0.9	22	23	0.25	0.39	0	25.2	0.7	582	39.2	8	42	0.22	3
46	0.17	0.09	1	23	34	0.35	0.38	0	31.9	0.7	554	52.2	6	34.8	0.2	0
924	0.05	0.08	0.6	3	74	0.37	0.08	0	48.1	1.4	384	24	0	34.7	0.13	0
995	0.16	0.09	1.1	34	176	0.34	0.16	0	52.7	1.1	530	31	9	49.6	0.16	0
18	0.05	0.26	0.7	31	79	0.23	0.13	0.9	187.2	0.5	447	20.8	39	117	0.08	0
67	0.06	0.03	0.8	28	100	0.25	0.08	0	25.2	0.5	216	14	11	30.8	0.11	0
56	0.1	0.36	0.5	13	2	0.05	0.15	0.6	272.9	1.1	609	25.5	26	176	0.05	3
37	0.25	0.45	0.2	41	4	0.25	0.02	0.6	334.2	0.6	469	32.8	68	289.1	0.06	4
520	0.2	0.36	0.5	27	29	0.79	0.11	0.5	252	1.1	482	33.8	52	227.3	0.14	2
3759	0.25	0.07	1.8	60	12	1.75	0.14	0	119	2.6	431	45.5	4	133	0.11	4
356	0.13	0.2	0.5	50	82	4.56	0.4	0.7	236.4	1	626	33.3	30	226.4	0.07	3
4189	0.23	0.08	1.7	27	3	0.46	0.19	0.4	65.3	3.1	737	69.1	4	222.7	0.31	8
7066	0.18	0	0.9	26	22	2.37	0.18	0	84	1.7	745	51.1	4	91.3	0.22	0
12617	0.12	0	0.4	18	17	1.38	0.15	0	49.8	0.6	334	14.7	3	38.1	0.06	3
45	0.17	0.1	0.6	38	10	4.3	0.14	0	106.6	1.8	777	75.7	0	185.8	0.24	0
2646	0.18	0.06	0.9	21	4	0.84	0.24	0	56.8	3.8	640	44.9	3	155.5	0.3	3
66	0.17	0.42	1.2	28	10	3.29	0.42	0.1	145.3	0.9	689	41.5	42	183.4	0.38	0
2530	0.3	0.07	3.4	71	79	4.24	0.48	0	40.9	1.8	844	29.8	7	107.9	0.11	4
77	0.23	0.13	0.8	54	30	2.85	0.4	0.4	157.5	1.2	827	40.2	17	201	0.1	3
5246	0.15	0.06	4.8	35	86	3.16	0.55	0	34.8	1.2	586	69.6	3	136.3	0.26	0
6	0.16	0.25	2.8	38	2	1.35	0.28	0	50.2	2	603	50.2	6	191.5	1.19	13
1286	0.13	0.03	0.4	23	19	3.36	0.23	0.1	106.6	1.4	359	19.4	3	64.6	0.06	0
385	0.11	0.03	0.8	34	10	2.59	0.17	0	56.2	1.8	540	36.5	3	81.5	0.25	3
8578	0.14	0	0.5	61	7	1.15	0.14	0	50.7	1	524	20.3	3	74.4	0.07	3
5427	0.13	0.04	0.9	13	42	0.9	0.17	5	116.1	2.7	843	77.4	22	279.5	0.43	17
136	0.28	0.28	2.4	42	11	1.36	0.52	1.7	272.6	1.3	1246	84.6	141	470	0.14	28
2718	0.14	0.17	4.3	20	22	0.58	0.38	0.8	34.1	2	522	34.1	7	221.7	0.24	10
88	0.48	0.2	3	8	11	0.12	0.24	1	48.1	1.9	686	32.1	4	224.6	0.08	12
2805	0.13	0.13	1.8	71	14	0.74	0.29	0.8	90.2	4.1	621	54.7	3	173.9	0.29	19
0	0	0	0	0	0	0	0	0	0	0	0	0	0	0	0	0
0	0	0	0	0	0	0	0	0	0	0	0	0	0	0	0	0
21087	0.22	0.03	0.5	22	16	1.75	0.35	0	47.7	0.7	452	9.5	3	38.2	0.06	3
32	0.09	0.06	0.4	6	17	1.12	0.18	0	20.6	0.4	388	14.7	0	32.3	0.09	0
67	0.13	0.05	0.5	22	16	1.05	0.13	0	56.5	0.6	549	10.8	0	37.7	0.05	3
12	0.09	0.06	0.6	15	58	0.9	0.15	0	17.5	0.4	265	11.6	6	29.1	0.09	0
12786	0.16	0.06	1.2	31	93	1.66	0.41	0	56.3	0.8	548	18.8	3	47	0.06	3

		Single portion	MAJOR NUTRIENTS								
Page	Description		Energy kcal	Protein g	Carbo- hydrate g	Sugars g	Fat g	Saturates g	Fibre g	Sodium mg	Salt g
81	Orange, plum and black grape	225	147	2.4	33.6	33.6	0.3	0	5.9	11	0.03
81	Orange, grape and ginger	210	144	2.8	32.5	31.8	0.4	0	5.8	13	0.03
82	Clementine, pineapple and cranberry	200	125	1.6	28.6	28.6	0.5	0	6.3	10	0.03
82	Clementine and cherry	195	125	2.7	27.7	27.7	0.3	0	5.9	10	0.03
83	Nectarine, apple and pineapple	200	182	4.2	40	40	0.5	0	7.6	6	0.02
83	Pear, grape and clementine	200	124	1.3	29.1	29.1	0.3	0	4.9	8	0.02
84	Pear, pineapple and grape	200	122	0.7	28.8	28.8	0.4	0	4.7	7	0.02
84	Pear, tomato and grapefruit	200	85	2	18.1	18.1	0.6	0.1	5.5	17	0.04
85	Pineapple and cherry	200	131	1.1	30.4	30.4	0.5	0	5.1	5	0.01
86	Pineapple, celery and watercress	170	85	1.8	17.5	17.5	0.9	0.1	4.0	68	0.17
86	Pineapple and ginger	210	145	0.5	34	33.7	0.7	0	4.3	8	0.02
87	Carrot, pineapple and ginger	215	142	1.1	32.4	31.6	0.9	0.1	6.8	35	0.09
87	Grapefruit, pineapple and clementine	200	135	1.8	30.6	30.6	0.5	0	5.3	10	0.03
88	Grape, apple and grapefruit	200	144	1.6	33.8	33.8	0.3	0	5.9	8	0.02
88	Plum, grape and beetroot	210	158	2.2	36.4	36.2	0.3	0	6	38	0.1
89	Plum, apple and pineapple juice	200	128	1	30	30	0.4	0	7	6	0.02
89	Pomegranate and pineapple	200	169	2.7	38	38	0.7	0	3.2	7	0.02
90	Melon, tomato and cucumber	190	50	2	9.4	9.4	0.5	0.1	3.6	23	0.06
90	Melon and red grape	200	101	1.4	23.3	23.3	0.3	0	3.2	15	0.04
91	Carrot, melon and cucumber	220	83	2.1	17.1	16.3	0.6	0.2	7	50	0.13
92	Tomato and orange	200	87	2.9	17.4	17.4	0.7	0.2	5.7	23	0.06
92	Tomato and plum	200	88	2.1	18.4	18.4	0.7	0.2	5.6	18	0.05
93	Tomato, beetroot and celery	200	61	2.7	10.8	10.5	0.8	0.2	5.1	88	0.22
93	Tomato, red pepper and carrot	220	91	2.5	17.8	17.1	1.1	0.3	7.4	51	0.13
94	**PARTY DRINKS**	ml									
94	Apple and lime zinger	70	32	0	8	8	0	0	0	0	0
94	Blackcurrant and coconut ripple	205	98	0.3	19.7	19.1	2	1.5	0	3	0.01
96	Clementini	125	55	0.7	13.1	12.9	0	0	0.3	3	0.01
96	Ginger lime fizz	280	24	0.1	6	6	0	0	0	1	0
97	Blue baby	90	71	1.8	15.8	15.8	0.1	0.1	1.4	33	0.08
97	Pink baby	100	35	1.8	7	7	0	0	0.2	33	0.08
98	Tequila bunrise	180	50	0.9	11.5	11.5	0	0	0.3	3	0.01
98	Pregna colada	165	96	0.7	15.6	14.7	3.5	3.5	0	13	0.03
99	Bun in the oven	175	65	0.2	16	16	0	0	2.1	1	0
99	Hot ginger and apple punch	266	136	0.1	33.8	33.6	0	0	0.1	2	0.01
100	**HOT DRINKS**	ml									
101	Chai masala	290	123	7	15.2	15	3.8	2.4	0.8	87	0.22
101	Spicy lemon	249	8	0.4	0.8	0.6	0.5	0.3	1	2	0.01
102	Spicy apple drink	260	89	0.2	21.4	21.4	0.2	0	0.7	5	0.01
103	Spiced milk	295	181	8.6	26.9	26.4	4.3	2.8	0.2	109	0.27
103	Swahili tea	289	114	6.9	13.9	13.9	3.5	2.2	0.3	86	0.22
104	White chocolate and raspberry drink	235	213	8.5	19.8	19.8	11.1	6.7	1	106	0.27
104	Chilli chocolate	295	175	12.6	14.4	13.4	7.4	4.6	3.7	234	0.59
105	Chocolate froth	220	187	8.2	19.1	17.6	8.7	5.4	0	94	0.24
108	**CORDIALS & COLD DRINKS**	ml									
108	Blackcurrant cordial	50	53	0.2	13.1	13.1	0	0	1	1	0
110	Lime cordial	50	85	0.1	20.7	20.7	0	0	0.1	1	0
111	Blueberry and lime cordial	50	52	0.3	12.5	11.2	0	0	1.1	0	0
112	Rhubarb cordial	50	71	0.4	18.6	18.6	0	0	0	4	0
113	Elderflower cordial	50	80	0	20.1	20.1	0	0	0	1	0
114	Ginger and lemongrass cordial	50	71	0.2	17.5	16.9	0.1	0.1	0.3	2	0.01
115	Fresh raspberry and apple drink	225	58	1.1	12.7	12.7	0.3	0.3	5.1	4	0.01
116	Fresh lemonade	125	117	0.9	27.7	27.7	0.3	0.3	4.4	6	0.02
117	Fresh orangeade	220	119	1.2	28.3	28.3	0.1	0.1	2.4	5	0.01
118	Iced tea	270	50	0.4	12.1	12.1	0	0	0.2	2	0.01
119	Pomegranate sherbet	50	59	0	14.7	14.7	0	0	0	1	0

	VITAMINS								MINERALS							
Carotene mcg	Thiamin mg	Riboflavin mg	Niacin mg	Folate mcg	Vitamin C mg	Vitamin E mg	Vitamin B6 mg	Vitamin B12 mcg	Calcium mg	Iron mg	Potassium mg	Magnesium mg	Iodine mcg	Phosphorus mg	Copper mg	Selenium mcg
387	0.23	0.1	1.7	46	79	0.81	0.29	0	87.8	0.8	627	26	3	65	0.29	3
117	0.25	0.09	1.1	63	108	0.47	0.32	0	107.4	0.6	562	31.6	6	63.2	0.22	3
147	0.28	0.11	0.9	35	103	0.14	0.28	0	77.2	0.8	484	42.1	0	45.6	0.21	0
196	0.23	0.1	0.9	46	135	0.1	0.2	0	81.8	0.4	461	29.4	0	58.9	0.07	0
343	0.18	0.13	2	4	118	0.49	0.22	0	40.1	1.4	703	44.5	9	75.7	0.27	4
89	0.14	0.08	0.6	17	47	0.53	0.17	0	44.6	0.6	444	19.5	3	41.9	0.17	0
48	0.14	0.08	0.7	8	20	0.65	0.17	0	39.5	0.6	457	28.2	3	33.8	0.25	0
738	0.19	0.06	1.7	57	63	2.13	0.22	0	41.3	0.9	646	22.3	3	60.4	0.06	0
62	0.19	0.1	0.9	16	36	0.32	0.23	0	51.8	0.6	528	42.1	0	38.9	0.29	0
1078	0.26	0.09	0.9	38	52	0.9	0.26	0	130.1	1.5	610	37.6	0	54.9	0.2	3
68	0.29	0.11	1.1	18	42	0.36	0.32	0	64.3	0.7	582	57.1	0	35.7	0.39	0
14889	0.33	0.07	1	26	36	0.92	0.4	0	73.2	0.9	608	43.9	4	43.9	0.29	0
107	0.26	0.11	1.1	55	104	0.41	0.26	0	81.2	0.6	616	44.3	0	55.4	0.22	0
42	0.16	0.06	0.6	29	45	0.81	0.23	0	42.1	0.6	557	22.7	0	48.6	0.16	3
627	0.14	0.07	2	78	13	0.95	0.24	0	47.7	1.5	846	27.3	0	85.3	0.34	0
267	0.16	0.06	1.1	6	18	1.44	0.22	0	28.3	0.6	465	25.1	0	37.7	0.19	0
95	0.22	0.15	1.1	80	46	0.18	0.73	0	54.6	1.7	735	47.3	0	72.8	0.51	0
3037	0.18	0.03	2.1	36	55	1.58	0.33	0	44.7	1.1	638	26.8	9	68.5	0.03	0
2809	0.11	0.05	1.2	11	45	0.16	0.3	0	46.6	0.8	575	24.7	8	41.1	0.14	0
21205	0.24	0.03	1.1	30	41	1.01	0.37	0	73.9	1	598	23.5	10	70.6	0.03	0
1014	0.32	0.06	2.3	83	112	2.41	0.39	0	83.5	1	648	25.7	6	73.8	0.1	0
1548	0.23	0.07	3.4	43	35	3.02	0.33	0	32.8	1.5	804	23	3	78.7	0.16	0
1163	0.22	0.03	2.2	146	41	2.55	0.31	0	46.7	1.8	893	24.9	3	90.2	0.03	0
19631	0.28	0.03	2.5	63	100	3.17	0.59	0	48.7	1.4	720	20.9	7	69.6	0.03	0
2	0	0	0	0	4	0	0.01	0	1.4	0	19	0.7	0	0.7	0.01	0
2	0	0	0	0	4	0	0.02	0	2.1	0	23	0	0	2.1	0.02	0
20	0.09	0.03	0.2	29	52	0.18	0.08	0	13.8	0.4	205	13.8	3	23.8	0.01	1
3	0	0	0	0	4	0	0.03	0	2.8	0	28	0	0	0	0.03	0
15	0.02	0.09	0.2	5	12	0	0.04	0	8.9	0.3	80	5.3	1	13.4	0.06	1
12	0.05	0.09	0.1	18	30	0.09	0.06	0	8.7	0.2	143	8.7	2	17.5	0.01	2
26	0.12	0.03	0.3	42	72	0.26	0.11	0	18	0.5	270	18	3	33	0	2
10	0.07	0.02	0.1	8	11	0.03	0.07	0	8.3	0.2	64	6.6	0	1.7	0.03	
11	0.02	0.02	0.1	2	6	0	0.04	0	5.3	0.4	47	3.5	0	5.3	0.02	0
3	0	0	0.1	0	0	0	0	0	0	0.1	19	2.7	0	2.7	0	0
26	0.06	0.5	0.3	21	4	0.09	0.12	1.8	252.8	1	362	29.4	59	194	0.03	3
12	0.02	0.1	0.1	5	12	0	0.02	0	14.9	1	67	7.5	0	7.5	0.05	0
5	0.03	0.03	0.3	8	15	0.16	0.05	0	15.6	0.3	252	10.4	0	15.6	0	0
27	0.09	0.59	0.4	24	5	0.09	0.18	2.2	303.9	0.2	428	32.5	74	239	0.03	3
17	0.06	0.49	0.2	20	4	0.09	0.12	1.8	242.8	1	350	26	61	190.7	0.03	3
19	0.07	0.49	0.3	24	9	0.14	0	0	244.4	0.1	338	25.9	61	0	0.02	2
242	0.12	0.74	0.6	30	6	0.18	0.18	2.7	374.7	1.2	637	85.6	91	351.1	0.38	3
18	0.07	0.48	0.2	18	4	0.09	0.11	1.8	240	0	312	22	59	187	0	2
20	0.01	0.01	0	0	20	0.2	0.01	0	13	0.3	74	3.5	0	8.5	0.04	0
1	0	0	0	0	6	0	0	0	3.4	0	17	1.5	0	1.5	0.03	0
1	0	0	0	0	2	0	0	0	1.5	0	7	0.5	0	0.5	0.01	0
25	0.03	0.1	0.1	3	2.5	0.1	0.01	0	42	0.1	127	6	0	7	0.05	0
1	0.01	0	0	2	2	0.01	0.01	0	2.5	0.1	10	1	0	1	0.03	0
6	0	0.01	0.1	0	1	0	0.02	0	4	0.1	41	4.5	0	4	0.02	0
5	0.02	0.05	0.5	29	38	0.36	0.07	0	24.8	0.6	239	20.3	0	29.3	0.07	0
17	0.05	0.04	0.2	0	55	0	0.1	0	83.1	0.5	143	12.4	0	17.4	0.27	1
31	0.11	0.04	0.5	33	57	0.26	0.11	0	50.4	0.2	166	11	2	21.9	0.07	2
11	0.05	0.05	0.1	27	29	0.08	0.05	0	8.2	0.2	180	10.9	0	19.1	0.03	0
7	0.01	0.01	0	0	2	0	0.06	0	2	0.1	41	1	0	1.5	0.03	0

INDEX

Recipes are listed under the name of their **main ingredient**; recipes listed in *italics* feature that ingredient in their title, although it is not their main ingredient.

ACKNOWLEDGEMENTS

I'd like to thank my family for their patience as this book unfolded and their helpful comments on the drinks, and concocting some great mocktail names, even if some were unpublishable!

Thanks also to Steve Taylor NMIMH Medical Herbalist for advice and reviewing the herbal drinks section. I am grateful to Lynne Waters, my dentist, for checking the section on sugars and sweeteners in pregnancy.

Picture Credits:
All images © Carroll & Brown with the exception of the following from Photolibrary.com: p2, p4, p13, p22, p33, p34 (background), p39, p45, p49, p59, p63, p64, p68, p74 (top), p92.

The author acknowledges the following references consulted in writing this book.

Adhami, V. M., N. Khan, et al (2009). 'Cancer chemoprevention by pomegranate: laboratory and clinical evidence.' *Nutr Cancer 61(6)*: 811-15.

British Soft Drinks Association (2010). *BSDA Code of Practice for High Caffeine Content Soft Drinks.*

Bates B, L. A., Swan G (2010). *National Diet and Nutrition Survey: Headline Results from Year 1 of the Rolling Programme (2008/2009)*. F. a. DH.

Berti C, et al (2010). 'Critical Issues in setting micronutrient recommendations for pregnant women: an insight.' *Maternal and Child Nutrition 6(Supp2)*: 5-22.

Cohen M (2007). 'Environmental toxins and health: the health impact of pesticides.' *Australian Family Physician 36(12)*.

European Commission: Nutrition Labelling Claims. Accessed Feb 2011 http://ec.europa.eu/food/food/labellingnutrition/claims/nutrition_claims_en.htm

D'Archivio, M., C. Filesi, et al (2007). 'Polyphenols, dietary sources and bioavailability.' *Ann Ist Super Sanita 43(4)*: 348-61.

Dangour, A. D., S. K. Dodhia, et al (2009). 'Nutritional quality of organic foods: a systematic review.'

Dangour, A. D., K. Lock, et al 'Nutrition-related health effects of organic foods: a systematic review.' *Am J Clin Nutr 92(1)*: 20310.

Dorling Kindersley (2010). *The Cook's Book of Ingredients.*

Duley, L., D. Henderson-Smart, et al (2005). 'Altered dietary salt for preventing pre-eclampsia, and its complications. *Cochrane Database Syst Rev(4)*: CD005548.

EFSA Panel on Dietetic Products Nutrition and Allergies (2010). *Scientific Opinion on Dietary Reference Values for Water*, EFSA 8.

Fischer-Rasmussen, W., S. K. Kjaer, et al (1991). 'Ginger treatment of hyperemesis gravidarum.' *Eur J Obstet Gynecol Reprod Biol 38(1)*: 19-24.

Gagne, A., S. Q. Wei, et al (2009). 'Absorption, transport, and bioavailability of vitamin E and its role in pregnant women.' *J Obstet Gynaecol Can 31(3)*: 210-17.

Gil, M. I., E. Aguayo, et al (2006). 'Quality changes and nutrient retention in fresh-cut versus whole fruits during storage. J Agric Food Chem 54(12)*: 4284-96.

GlaxoSmithKline (2010). *Acid erosion: causes, signs and prevention.*

Granado, F., B. Olmedilla, et al (1996). 'Major fruit and vegetable contributors to the main serum carotenoids in the Spanish diet.' *Eur J Clin Nutr 50(4)*: 246-50.

Hajslova, J., V. Schulzova, et al (2005). 'Quality of organically and conventionally grown potatoes: four-year study of micronutrients, metals, secondary metabolites, enzymic browning and organoleptic properties. *Food Addit Contam 22(6)*: 514-34.

Harland, J. (2007). 'Soya Isoflavones and their effect on the hormone milieu.' *Complete Nutrition 7(2)*.

Hartmann, A., C. D. Patz, et al (2008). 'Influence of processing on quality parameters of strawberries.' *J Agric Food Chem 56(20)*: 9484-9.

Hofmeyr, G. J., T. A. Lawrie, et al 'Calcium supplementation during pregnancy for preventing hypertensive disorders and related problems.' *Cochrane Database Syst Rev(8)*: CD001059.

Holst, L., D. Wright, et al (2009). 'The use and the user of herbal remedies during pregnancy.' *J Altern Complement Med 15(7)*: 787-92.

Jahanfar, S. and H. Sharifah (2009). 'Effects of restricted caffeine intake by mother on fetal, neonatal and pregnancy outcome.' *Cochrane Database Syst Rev(2)*: CD006965.

Kilpatrick, S. J. and K. L. Safford (1993). 'Maternal hydration increases amniotic fluid index in women with normal amniotic fluid.' *Obstet Gynecol 81(1)*: 49-52.

Kramer, M. S. and R. Kakuma (2003). Energy and protein intake in pregnancy.' *Cochrane Database Syst Rev(4)*: CD000032.

Mahomed, K., Z. Bhutta, et al (2007). 'Zinc supplementation for improving pregnancy and infant outcome.' *Cochrane Database Syst Rev(2)*: CD000230.

Marti, N., P. Mena, et al (2009). 'Vitamin C and the role of citrus juices as functional food.' *Nat Prod Commun 4(5)*: 677-700.

McKillop, D. J., K. Pentieva, et al (2002). 'The effect of different cooking methods on folate retention in various foods that are amongst the major contributors to folate intake in the UK diet.' *Br J Nutr 88(6)*: 681-8.

Pellegrini, N., E. Chiavaro, et al 'Effect of different cooking methods on color, phytochemical concentration, and antioxidant capacity of raw and frozen brassica vegetables.' *J Agric Food Chem 58(7)*: 4310-21.

Roe, M. *Vitamin Losses in Smoothies.* Institute of Food Research Norwich (personal communication January 2011)

Rumbold, A. and C. A. Crowther (2005). 'Vitamin C supplementation in pregnancy.' *Cochrane Database Syst Rev(2)*: CD004072.

Scientific Advisory Committee on Nutrition (2010). Iron and Health. *S. A. C. o. Nutrition*, The Stationery Office.

Strobel, M., J. Tinz, et al (2007). 'The importance of beta-carotene as a source of vitamin A with special regard to pregnant and breastfeeding women.' *Eur J Nutr 46 Suppl 1*: I1-20.

Sultana, S., F. A. Ripa, et al 'Comparative antioxidant activity study of some commonly used spices in Bangladesh.' *Pak J Biol Sci 13(7)*: 340-3.

Tarozzi, A., S. Hrelia, et al (2006). 'Antioxidant effectiveness of organically and non-organically grown red oranges in cell culture systems.' *Eur J Nutr 45(3)*: 152-8.

Thaver, D., M. A. Saeed, et al (2006). 'Pyridoxine (vitamin B6) supplementation in pregnancy.' *Cochrane Database Syst Rev(2)*: CD000179.

United Kingdom Tea Council: 'Tea and antioxidant properties.' Fact Sheet. Accessed Feb 2011

Weed, S. (1986). *Wise Woman Herbal for the Childbearing Year.* Ash Tree Publishing.

Williamson, C. S. (2006). *Nutrition in Pregnancy.* British Nutrition Foundation.

Wunderlich, S. M., C. Feldman, et al (2008). 'Nutritional quality of organic, conventional, and seasonally grown broccoli using vitamin C as a marker.' *Int J Food Sci Nutr 59(1)*: 34-45.